The Goldilocks Principle

A PRACTICAL GUIDE
TO THE CHAKRAS

Teri Leigh

TeriLeigh LLC

TeriLeigh LLC
www.terileigh.com

Book Layout ©2013 BookDesignTemplates.com

Ordering Information:
Quantity sales. Special discounts are available on quantity purchases by corporations, associations, and others. For details, contact the "Special Sales Department" at the address above.

Disclaimer
This publication contains the ideas and opinions of the author and is intended to provide helpful and informative material based on the author's personal experience and knowledge. It is sold with the understanding that the author is not engaged in providing medical, health, or other professional services. Readers should consult professional medical, health and other professionals before participating in any of the practices suggested in this book. The author disclaims all responsibility for liability, loss or risk which is incurred by readers' use and application of any of the contents of this book.
Printed in the United States of America
First Printing: October 2012

The Goldilocks Principle: A Practical Guide to the Chakras. Teri Leigh. —1st ed.
ISBN 978-0-9559643-3-7

To my ancestors,
Grandpa Edgar and Grandma Alice,
for teaching me how to laugh and cry
and reminding me that you are in my bones.

Table of Contents

The Goldilocks Principle describes a situation that is "just right" rather than too much or not enough.

CHAPTER ONE

Introduction

The Story of the Three Bears

Once upon a time, a curly haired blonde girl named Goldilocks, happened across a cottage in the woods. The cottage belonged to three bears, who prided themselves on creating a homey and loving environment. As they were good and responsible bears, they left their porridge to cool on the table whilst they went for their morning walk to enjoy the sunshine and fresh air of the beautiful day.

Goldilocks, on the other hand, was having a rough morning. She had not slept well the night before because her mother and father were up arguing all night long. When Goldilocks asked her mother for breakfast, her mother told her she was a very bad girl for always needing things that she didn't have to give and kicked her out of the house for the day. Poor Goldilocks went wandering in the woods, feeling tired, hungry, and rather defeated.

The three bears were rather trusting creatures and had left their door unlocked and their windows open. The smell of cooling porridge on the table coaxed Goldilocks into the kitchen where she found three bowls. She first tried the porridge in the largest bowl, which belonged to Papa Bear. It tasted nice, but she spit it out quickly as it was too hot. Then, she tried the porridge in the medium bowl, which belonged to Mama Bear. She swallowed that porridge with a grimace as it was too cold. The porridge in the smallest bowl, which belonged to Baby Bear, was just right, making her feel warm inside with every bite, so she ate it all.

Because the house was so inviting and she felt somewhat safe and comfortable there after having taken in the nourishment from the porridge, Goldilocks ventured into the living room where she found three chairs. She first sat in the largest chair, and imagined herself as the king of the household. Although the chair made her feel bigger and stronger, she quickly got up because it was too hard. Then she tried the medium sized chair which made her feel gentle, but climbed out because it was too soft. Finally, she sat in the third and smallest chair, which was just right because it felt like the perfect balance between strong and gentle.

Goldilocks felt much better than she had when she left her own home that morning, and she ventured upstairs to the bedroom where she found three beds. Having had so little sleep the night before, the beds called to her. She first tried the largest bed. It was so large that it made her feel like she was important, but she found it too hard. Then she tried the medium bed, which was so cozy that it made her feel special, but it was too soft. Finally, she curled up in the smallest bed, which was just right. She quickly fell into a deep sleep of happy dreams.

When the bears returned from their walk, Papa Bear and Mama Bear sat down to his porridge and discovered it had been tasted while Baby Bear said, "Someone's eaten my porridge all up! That's okay, because I'm full from the berries I had on the walk anyway."

They retreated to their living room, and Papa and Mama Bear discovered their chairs had been moved as if they had been sat in. Baby Bear discovered his chair to have cracked slightly under the weight of Goldilocks and said, "Someone's been rocking in my chair and broke it! That's okay, I am about to outgrow this one anyway."

Curious as to what else had been disturbed in their cottage, they went up to the bedroom. Papa and Mama Bear discovered their bedsheets to be disheveled as if someone had slept in them, and Baby Bear found Goldilocks still asleep in his bed. "Someone's been sleeping in my bed, and she's still there! That's okay because I'm not tired right now anyway." So, the three bears tiptoed downstairs to finish their breakfast and go about their day.

The Goldilocks Principle

Definition

The Goldilocks Principle describes a situation that is "just right" rather than too much or not enough. This ideology is derived from the popular children's story and has been applied to many disciplines, including astronomy, biology, psychology, economics, and more. In astronomy, a Goldilocks Planet is one that is just the right distance from a star to be able to sustain life on the planet. In ecomonics, a Goldilocks Economy sustains moderate growth and low inflation. In cognitive science or education, the Goldilocks Principle is observed when a task is neither too simple nor too complex for the learner to grasp. In medicine, The Goldilocks Principle is the ideal dosage of a drug for a particular patient based on their physiological needs. In each of these examples, optimal balance "just right" is attained.

This slightly adapted version of "The Story of the Three Bears" depicted above is a perfect case study of the Goldilocks Principle as it applies to overall health and wellness, both physiologically and energetically. Each item in the cottage symbolizes a situation in Goldilocks's life that is operating within an extreme. The porridge provides physical nourishment when she is hungry, and energetic nurturing that she misses from her own parents. The chairs provide a sense of self as she "takes her seat." The beds provide both physical rest and sleep as well as a sense of peace which is lacking in her own home. As she finds "just right" with the item, she discovers a state of "just right" within herself. Symbolically, the item serves as the medicine for a particular physical or energetic ailment in her life. Just as a doctor is considered on some levels a healer, the food, home, and energy of the bears in the cottage of this adaptation of the story is what heals

Goldilocks of her ailments by bringing her to a state of equilibrium akin to The Goldilocks Principle.

Energy is Contagious

Goldilocks learned that energy is contagious. Goldilocks left home that morning having contracted the energetic dis-ease of scarcity. She was hungry, tired, and defeated. The bear's cottage held the energy of peace. The nurturing and loving environment left Goldilocks feeling safe, nourished, and supported.

The adage "misery loves company" supports the concept that energy is contagious. For example, if you are in a good mood and you walk into a room of people who have just received some very bad news, it doesn't take long for you to feel the misery of the room without them even telling you the news. Or the opposite may occur, you may be in a really bad mood and walk into a room of happy people, and pretty soon, they are cheering you up and you are feeling better. Their energy is contagious to you, and you walk away feeling better and your mood may calm their giddiness.

Thus, through her ventures in the cottage in the woods, Goldilocks learned the valuable spiritual lesson of "be careful the company you keep" because the people and energies of the people with whom you engage is contagious to your own life. At this particular time of her life, the energy of her parents was causing dis-ease for Goldilocks, whereas the energy of the three bears provided necessary medicine to treat her dis-ease and bring her to a more optimal experience of life.

Everything is Connected

The reason energy is contagious is because everything is connected, constantly sharing the same energy. Perhaps on an unconscious level, all the characters in the story instinctively knew that all living beings are sharing energy all the time and thus made the circumstances available to share with each other. Goldilocks felt compelled to enter the cottage in the woods that houses all the things she needed. At the same time, the bears were trusting enough to leave their doors and windows open and available for her to enter. Goldilocks made herself at home in the bears' cottage as if the items in the cottage weren't owned or possessed by anyone, but were there for anyone who may need them. Just as many indigenous tribes do not believe in ownership or possessing of land or items, this story emphasizes the power of sharing and supporting each other because everything is connected.

On one level, all living beings share energy as a means of mutually supporting one another, symbolic of the ultimate balance of the universe. For example, when a predator kills its prey, the energy contained in its body is not destroyed, but rather it is transmitted to the predator and scavengers and serves as fuel for the living. Then, the carcass that remains decomposes into the ground and is fed on by various insects, worms, grubs and maggots. The excrement of all the creatures that eat of the corpse then gets absorbed by the soil and serves as fertilizer for plants to grow, which in turn feeds other animals and creatures on the planet, keeping everything in cycle. This simple ecosystem example just shows how energy is constantly moving and changing to support the balance and well-being of the entire system.

In the modern world, the same is the case within a community. Each person provides his or her talents to the rest of the community. The doctors, the teachers, the homemakers, the builders, the scientists, the historians, the mathematicians, the coaches, the politicians, etcetera, all mutually support each other, each giving something the others need, while at the same time having their own needs provided by others.

The three bears were trusting and loving enough to leave their doors and windows open, and thus Goldilocks was able to be supported by them while they were out in the woods getting their exercise having their own needs met by the forest. In this version of the story, Baby Bear understood the needs of Goldilocks and surrendered to her willingly because he trusted that when the time came, his needs would be met somehow as hers had been.

On another level, everything is connected because it is all made up of the same stuff. Although unconsciously, perhaps the bears left their doors open to Goldilocks because had she knocked on their door in search of nourishment and support, they would have openly given to her because they hold compassion for any living being whose needs are not met. Whether they have gone hungry and needy before or not, their muscles and tissues are made of the same energy as hers and they can relate on a cellular level to the plight of being in need.

On the cellular level, everything in the world is made up of a collection of particles. In high school chemistry classes, students learn to balance chemical equations by calculating how molecules are reconfiguring themselves. Put simply, molecules and atoms (particles) are constantly "jumping ship" from one to another. For example, when you exhale, the breath that escapes your lips is made up of various molecules that you carried within your system for a span of time. Then someone in your vicinity may inhale those same molecules, which then blend and reorganize themselves with the other molecules they carry around in their body. If you consider that molecules carry energy, then you are constantly sharing energy with all living beings that breathe air.

The law of physics known as "the law of conservation of energy" that was first formulated in the nineteenth century states that energy can change its location and its form, but it can neither be created nor destroyed. Thus, particles that contain energy may change their shape and their form and "jump ship" from one object or being to another, but the energy contained within the particles is never created nor destroyed, it just moves around and shape-shifts.

Goldilocks and the bears lived within walking distance of each other's home, so it can be assumed that they were constantly exchanging energy, not only through the air they breathed, but through the molecules and particles in their food they ate that was harvested from the same plants in the woods. While Goldilocks had a home of her own, the bears' cottage provided something energetically unseen yet vital to her equilibrium of health and wellness. She entered because her cells knew that what she needed was inside. Some things needed and provided within the ecosystem or community are physical and concrete, such as food and shelter, while other things needed and provided are energetic, such as love and nurturing. In this story, Goldilocks's own home was not loving and nurturing at the time, and in the case of food, it did not provide nourishment either. On the other hand, the bears' cottage had an abundance of love, nourishment, food, and warmth to provide, so it did. In fact, Baby Bear felt so supported that when he discovered Goldilocks in his bed, he let her stay there to get the rest she needed because he had already had enough.

On the surface, this story appears to depict how Goldilocks had her physical needs of hunger and exhaustion met by the porridge and beds of the bears. However, on a deeper level, she was also provided with non-physical needs of nurturing and love. The cycle of sharing of energy was maintained on multiple levels because where the bears received both physical and non-physical nourishment and support from the fresh air of the woods on their walk, Goldilocks received both physical and non-physical nourishment and support from the welcoming and inviting cottage.

The world consists of both a harmonious and natural physical world as well as an invisible energetic realm which are intricately connected. While the physical world includes all things you can see, feel, smell, hear, and touch, the spiritual world includes all things you can imagine, know, and believe. Just as your physical body has tissues and bones, your energetic body has thoughts and emotions. Your thoughts and emotions directly impact your physical sensations and experiences. At the same time, your physical sensations and experiences can directly impact your thoughts and emotions. For example, As Goldilocks physically felt hungry, the pangs in her stomach resulted in an emotional state of fear or anxiety that led her to trespass. On the flip side, the feelings of love and nurturing that Baby Bear felt from his parents and environment resulted in a physical feeling of nourishment and strength which meant he didn't need more food or rest, even after a walk in the woods. The physical and the energetic are both part of the whole. Like the construction of a spider web, the empty space between the threads is just as important as the physical threads themselves.

Like the ecosystem or a community, your body serves as an interconnected system of contagious energy. You have a physical body and an energetic body that intertwine and influence each other. Your bones, tissues, muscles, organs, etc. make up your physical anatomy, and your chakras, nadis, and your aura all make up your energetic anatomy. The physical and energetic integrate to create the whole.

The Goldilocks Effect

When the physical and non-physical systems of your being integrate and work together, what results is the concept of finding "just right." In the story, Baby Bear's system was supported physically and energetically, so much so that he could provide that energy to Goldilocks when she needed it. While **The Goldilocks Principal** is the concept of finding "just right," **The Goldilocks Effect** is what results when "just right" is found.

We've all experienced The Goldilocks Effect at various times in our lives. Although perhaps fleeting, these times are when we feel physically healthy and emotionally balanced and everything in life seems to work out "just right." These moments may be just that, moments, like when you performed well at a task or felt "in the zone." Sometimes, these moments may last longer, like when you are happiest in a particular job and home or most fulfilled by the experiences of our lives. Ultimately, The Goldilocks Effect is not something that is attained from external forces or outside environments or factors, but rather, it is a result of the internal balance of the physical and non-physical energies of your being.

Finding "Just Right" as a Collective

Although "Just Right" is an internal state of being, it can be influenced somewhat by the external, particularly by the

13

contagious energy of those around you. The nourishment and nurturing provided by the bears' cottage to Goldilocks impacted how Goldilocks ultimately felt inside herself. However, she had to be open to receiving the nourishment the cottage and the bears provided. If she had never entered the cottage and imbibed of its energy, her internal state may not have been altered.

Energy is contagious, and when you are surrounded by certain energies, they can affect you dramatically as a collective. If you practice yoga, you may have experienced this concept when you were part of a large class or were assisted by a talented instructor. In a large yoga class you naturally borrow energy from the other students and you may feel stronger and more flexible that you are naturally or when you practice yoga by yourself. The same is true when you are assisted by a talented instructor. You may find that you can perform a pose at a significantly deeper intensity of strength and flexibility with even a gentle touch of an instructor than you can without their aid because they are lending you their energy for the pose.

The following experiment is an example of The Goldilocks Effect occurs as a result of collective energies merging. It also demonstrates the power of energy and interconnectedness on the physical form, like an ecosystem. The following levitation experiment is an example of how five people can create the Goldilocks Effect together.

One person sits in a chair while four other people stand around him. These four people form their hands like guns, interlaced fingers with released index fingers, each one taking their extended fingers (right up to the fist) into the armpit or knee-pit of the man in the chair. They attempt to lift the man from the chair using just their fingers. Inevitably, they struggle with his weight.

Then, one by one, each of the four places their right hands and then their left hands, without touching each other, over the head of the man in the chair, stacking hand upon hand into a tower of eight hands above his head. Some participants may feel something energetically such as tingling, vibration, heat, or chills. More often than not, one of the people standing has a very grounded energy while another one has a light and airy energy, like feathers, another one has a more flowing energy, while another is more still. Each energy is different, sometimes appearing quite opposite to the others, but they always blend nicely. While one person may provide the energy of earth through stability, another may provide the energy of water through movement, another may provide the energy of air through lightness, and so forth. After a few moments of holding their hands over the man's head they each to remove their hands from his head and try to lift him again, the same as before. This time, they lift him with ease, usually at least to shoulder height.

Earlier, you learned that energy is contagious. In this experiment, the energy of each individual in the group is contagious to each other. They share and blend their energies to create an optimal whole, creating the Goldilocks Effect of "just right" and proving that everything is connected. This small group of people has become an ecosystem complete with water, earth, air, fire, and more, mutually supporting each other in the whole. They are no longer separate, but one unit working together.

This experiment is an example of how the energetic system of the body serve to support the physical function of the body in balance and energy. The person seated has an energy center at the crown of his head that receives the energy from the energy centers in the palms of the hands of the other four people. At the same time, the energy centers of each person being stacked in this way allows the energy to transmit through all five people, linking them together as one whole unit rather than five separate beings. When they all unite as one, the process of lifting becomes easier as they are balanced with stability, strength, lightness, and grace.

If the person seated in the chair, or any individual person in the collective is non-receptive to the energy transmission, the experiment is not as successful and The Goldilocks Effect is not achieved. Ultimately, The Goldilocks Effect comes from within.

Finding "Just Right" as an Individual

While it is helpful and useful to borrow energy from others to get tastes and feelings of The Goldilocks Effect, ideally, you would not be dependent on others to provide the energy you need, but rather, you learn how to reorganize the energy within your own system to its optimal balance.

In "The Story of the Three Bears" Goldilocks was dependent upon the energy of the bears and their cottage to provide the balance she needed. If she continues to rely on them to provide what she needs, the situation could easily devolve into a scenario that can be likened to a drug addict's (Goldilocks) relationship to her dealer (the bears). Like the proverb "give a man a fish, he eats of a day; teach a man to fish, he eats for a lifetime," the bears would be best off teaching Goldilocks how to ultimately nourish and nurture herself.

This book is a practical guide to understanding the interconnectedness between your physical body and your energetic system. After gaining an understanding of how the two systems intertwine, you will learn the characteristics and qualities of the different energy centers of your body (chakras) as well as simple and practical physical techniques you can apply to adjust and calibrate the energy within your chakras in order to find "just right" for yourself.

CHAPTER TWO

Energetic Systems

Introduction

Because everything is connected, and energy is contagious, applying the Goldilocks Principle to both your physical and energetic bodies is healing on all levels: physical, mental, emotional, psychological, spiritual, and more. This chapter explains how the physical and the energetic systems of your body work together to provide a full human experience.

You have a physical body comprised of fluids that travel through vessels, process in organs, and produces actions and expressions through tissues and muscles. Layered inside and around the physical body is an energetic body comprised of life force energy. This life force energy travels through energy channels called *nadis*, processes in energy centers called *chakras*, and produces expressions through energy fields called *auras*. The physical and energetic bodies work congruently and intricately with each other.

Let's define your life force as your *essence,* that part of you that is not your body and not your thoughts, but is your *soul.* Your essence, your soul experiences life in the physical world through the human body. Your body is the vehicle and expressive container of your life force. The energy of the human body can be compared to an electronic device. Your muscles, tissues, and organs make up the physical body, the hardware. Your thoughts, ideas, and emotions make up the mind, the software. Maintaining a healthy physical body is just like keeping the hardware of your device in proper working order. If a wire gets frayed, or the screen gets broken, the device doesn't function as well. If you break a bone or injure a muscle, your body doesn't function as well. Similarly, if your device is overloaded with software, or your software has bugs, the device doesn't work as well. If your mind is cluttered or confused, your experience of life is also cluttered and confused.

Another analogy to understand the anatomy (form) and physiology (function) of the energetic body is to compare it to a lamp. The human life force is the electricity itself. The life force (electricity) travels through the body through energy channels called *nadis*, like the wires of the lamp. At certain points throughout the body, the life force energy gathers into energy centers called *chakras*, like the light bulbs of the lamp. The *chakras* process the energy and produce an energy field called an *aura*, like the light from a light bulb. Without the electricity, the lamp is just a collection of wires, bulbs, and other matter that has the potential to create light. Without life force energy, the human body is just a collection of tissues, organs, bones, and channels with nothing moving through them.

From the physical perspective, clinical death is when the heart stops pumping and the lungs stop breathing. The actions of the heart and lungs are controlled by the autonomic nervous system in the brain. Therefore, if your brain, heart, or lungs stop working, the eventual result is death. From an energetic perspective, death is when the life force leaves the human body. This occurs when the chakras (energy centers) stop moving energy, they shut off, or close completely.

The Systems of the Body

The Brain - Nervous System - Electricity

From a physiological standpoint, the electrical system of the human body is the nervous system, controlled by the brain and spinal cord.

When you have a thought that you would like to move a part of your body, your brain sends the message along the spinal cord and nerves to the muscles that control that body part. In the reverse, if a body part receives a message about the external world, a smell, for example, the message is sent from the body part along the nerves to the brain where the mind interprets the information, in this case, identifying the smell. A healthy nervous system keeps clear communication channels through the nerves and the spinal cord to the brain. If the channels are not clear or get mixed up, just like wires getting crossed in an old-fashioned telephone circuit board, the messages can be confused. The brain must be able to clearly interpret and respond to the information that travels on the nervous system. If the information is mis-perceived or mis-understood, just like in the childhood game of telephone, the appropriate responses are not likely to be delivered.

Again, the mind-body connection is vital to optimal experience. The mind must appropriately process the information provided and effectively communicate the response messages to the body, and the body must transmit these messages efficiently through its channels.

The Heart - Circulatory System - Plumbing

Another way to understand how energy functions in your body is to understand the movement of energy through your body like blood and lymphatic fluids move through the fluid systems of your body. Your circulatory system consists of millions of little pipes and tubes called arteries, veins, vessels and capillaries, to transport fluid around your body. The capillaries are the tiniest of blood vessels, small enough to transport single cells of blood. Each vessel, vein, artery, and capillary is like one *nadi* (energy channel). Each intersection of a channel with another is a *chakra*. For as many times as blood vessels and veins, even tiny single-cell-sized capillaries intersect with each other in the body, you have that many chakras. Thus, you have upwards of 72 million *chakras*.

Your lymph system has nodes, little pockets (or discs) of juice that filter the lymphatic fluid from the lymphatic vessels and veins into the bloodstream. These nodes are housed mostly in your armpits, groin, chest, and neck, where veins and vessels intersect. The lymphatic system does not have a heart-like pump to move the lymph fluid. It depends upon movement of your body to pump the fluid throughout your system. Body movement, gravity, muscle compression and release of the lymph nodes (like squeezing a toothpaste tube) move the lymphatic fluid through your system. Each lymph node, pocket or disc of juice, houses a *chakra*.

The energetic system of your body works very similarly to the fluid systems of your body. The major chakras, somewhat like the human heart, function as large pumps to actively move energy through your system. The smaller minor chakras right down to the smallest of chakra serve like lymph nodes, filtering the energy.

Should you receive acupuncture, the needles are placed into chakras along the energy lines of your body to assist in the flow of energy within those channels. Just like your veins and arteries, energy lines can get clogged, limiting the flow. The needles help redirect the energy flow, like directing traffic, to serve to clear those clogs. Placed into the more major chakras, the needles can aid in jumpstarting the pulsation of the chakra, much like CPR massages the heart to facilitate circulation. Some acupuncturists even use electrical impulses attached to the needles for this purpose. Acupressure works in a similar way, compressing the chakras (like compressing lymph nodes) to move energy through the energy channels called meridians.

Just as physical exercise of any form supports the circulatory system by working the heart and lymph nodes to move blood and lymphatic fluid through your body, physical exercise also supports the energetic system by working the chakras to move energy through your system. In particular, exercise such as yoga, tai chi, and qigong are specifically designed to work the chakras and move energy through the system for optimal functioning. Exercise is simply a process of maintaining a healthy system for your body, both physically and energetically.

The Lungs - Respiratory System -Ventilation

Your life force energy doesn't only travel through the nervous system and the circulatory system, but also through the respiratory system. Breath is vital to the physical functioning of the body and probably has the most immediate impact on your non-physical experiences (your thoughts and emotions). Whenever you are distraught or stressed, a few deep breaths usually suffices to calm both your mind and body.

On a physiological level, when you breathe, the air goes into your lungs, which filter the air and send it directly to your heart. The air attaches to blood cells in the lung and is then pumped to the various tissues, muscles, organs, and bones throughout your body. In addition, deep breathing, especially through your nose, hits certain ganglia and nerve endings that trigger your nervous system to send messages to your brain to slow down your heart rate, lower your blood pressure, and provide calm. Rapid breathing, on the other hand, stimulates the nervous system to kick into fight or flight mode and send hormones into your system to speed up your heart rate and increase your blood pressure. Thus, how you breathe tells your body, through your nervous system, how it needs to function for the particular activities it needs to perform.

Blood and lymph are the physical liquids that carry oxygen to the muscles and tissues throughout the body. The oxygen is carried in the blood to the muscles and tissues where it serves as the fuel for the actions that the muscles and tissues perform. The respiratory system is in essence, the ventilation of your system, creating space and room for everything in your system to move. When you get tense, your muscles tighten and constrict, limiting the expression of your body through lowered range of motion, less space. The air that travels through the pipes and tubes of your body, both physically and energetically, creates space for things to occur, ventilation.

The nervous system is the electrical system of your body; and the circulatory system is the plumbing of your body, and your respiratory system is the ventilation system of your body. Your "wires and circuit boards" as well as your "pipes and pumps" and your "fans and ducts" need to be kept in proper working condition both physically and energetically. The state of your physical body is a direct reflection of the efficiency of energy flow through your energetic body and vice versa. Both your physical body your energetic body, the hardware and software respectively of your body need to be maintained for optimal functioning and fullness of the human experience. Herein lies the importance of the mind-body connection.

Unlike the smart-phone with the broken screen or the computer with a virus, we cannot trade-in our broken bodies when they wear out, or upgrade to a newer model when our mind gets 'fried'. Instead, we pay doctors, nutritionists, and fitness trainers to tend to the hardware of our bodies. We pay therapists, teachers, and other information experts to tend to the software of our minds. These professionals and the services they recommend come at a premium cost of time, money, and effort. Thus, we often choose to forgo the recommended check-ups and maintenance routines, at which point we can quickly find ourselves playing the game of multiple medications. Some medications are used to counteract the side effects of others. Quite often, medications merely mask symptoms and do not treat the underlying issues. Medication addresses issues solely from a physiological perspective, providing chemicals, hormones, or other physical compounds, but completely ignore treatment of the issue from a mindfulness and energetic approach.

In order to diagnose and treat imbalances that create discomfort or disease, you must first understand the integration of the physical with the energetic and then determine how to integrate your maintenance and treatment of the two systems as one. When the physical body and energetic body are integrated and in balance,

The Goldilocks Effect results, causing a state of equilibrium and homeostasis.

Homeostasis

Homeostasis is the ability of the body (physical and energetic integrated as one unit) to assess external conditions and adjust appropriately in order to maintain a condition of equilibrium or stability internally.

In our story, the external conditions of Goldilocks's home were so severe that they negatively impacted her internal state. The lack of proper rest and food compounded with the tension between her parents and the emotional stress of being yelled at by her mother, Goldilocks's internal equilibrium was unable to appropriately compensate and she was left in a state of imbalance and dis-ease. She was not living in her body in a state of homeostasis, energetically or physically.

The three bears, on the other hand, had developed a healthy diet of proper rest, healthy nutrition, loving environment, and interaction with the natural world around them to support homeostasis. Thus, when an imbalanced external force (Goldilocks) entered their environment, they were able to adjust accordingly and not be distraught or disturbed by her presence. In fact, Baby Bear's system was so healthy that when he recognized a need for increased energy of love, nourishment, and rest, his system was able to process it as necessary and share it with Goldilocks.

If we were to continue the story, perhaps Baby Bear would offer to become a sort of personal trainer and life coach for Goldilocks, teaching her how to take care of her physical body and provide for her energetic needs herself. Any doctor or nurse will attest to the fact that a positive attitude supports healing better than a negative one, and that patients respond better when surrounded by happy loved ones than when left alone or surrounded by sourpusses. Goldilocks stumbled upon some very potent natural and energetic medicine when she came across the bears' cottage. At least for that day, and perhaps more in the future, she could treat the virus of sourpuss parents with the antidote of the happy bears.

The good news is that physical and energetic homeostasis is something that can be taught and learned, as well as something that can be shared with others. Perhaps one day Goldilocks can learn how to access and attune her own internal calibrators to achieve homeostasis without becoming dependent on the medicine of the bears.

CHAPTER THREE

The Chakras

Introduction

Definitions

Chakra*: a disc shaped energy center that regulates, filters, and radiates energy through channels. The "lightbulb" of your energetic lamp.*

Nadi*: an energy channel, also known as a meridian, through which energy is transmitted from one part of the body to another. The "wires" of your energetic lamp.*

Aura*: the radiant multi-colored, multi-faceted energy that appears as colored light that emits beyond the physical body of the living being. The "light" emitting from your energetic lamp.*

When doctors assess your physical health, their first concern is your vital signs, which basically give them a general picture of the functioning of your heart, lungs, and brain, the three areas discussed in depth in Chapter 2. In the same way, the concern of this book is with the main "organs" of the energetic body which are the seven major chakras: root, sacral, core, heart, throat, third eye, and crown.

Qualities

The chakras are depicted as colors and light. While this depiction is accurate, it is incomplete. Chakras actually hold many different qualities. Cardiologists use many characteristics to assess the state of a human heart, including the sound and rate of the beat, the volume of blood pumped, the texture of the muscle, the color and density of the tissue, the size and shape of the organ, and more. Furthermore, the health of the heart is influenced by many factors including lifestyle, genetics, environment, illness or disease, and more. The following lists are not exhaustive, but give an idea of how multi-faceted the chakras are:

Chakra Qualities	
Characteristics	**Influences**
Color	Childhood Development
Density	Genetics
Shape	Tragedies & Traumas
Size	Triumphs & Successes
Texture	Environment
Movement	Nutrition & Diet
Vibration	Exercise & Fitness
Tone	Friends & Family
Sound	Career
Volume	Stress Factors
Temperature	Personality
Imagery	Likes & Preferences
Brightness	Aversions
	Gifts & Talents
	Hobbies
	Spirituality & Religion
	Relationships
	Past experiences
	Future hopes & dreams

Each of these characteristics adjusts in its own way to address external circumstances and influences as they arise. How the chakra develops and is influenced by circumstances in your life somewhat determines how it will adjust to address future circumstances.

Like a muscle, the chakra develops based on both how you are genetically coded and how much you work the chakra. While some people are born into genetics that are muscularly stronger and others are born into genetics that are muscularly more flexible, you are born into genetic coding of your chakras as well. While the muscularly strong person can stretch their muscles to create more flexibility, they may never be as limber as the muscularly flexibly person and vice versa. The same applies to your chakras.

Just as the water pressure and temperature in a plumbing system can be turned up and down, or a light bulb can be dimmed or brightened, a chakra can be tuned as well. Think of the chakras like muscles that can be worked at different levels depending upon the amount of effort exerted to create the necessary amount of force. A healthy chakra is one that can appropriately create just the right amount of force, tune itself to the right temperature, pressure, brightness, vibration, and so forth, according to the circumstance. For example, there will be times in your life where you will need more compassion from your heart chakra versus other times in your life when you will need more personal power from your core chakra. A healthy chakra system can adjust and compensate accordingly.

In addition, chakras serve as sort of storage houses for life force energy, and share and trade energy between and among themselves as necessary to adjust to external circumstances. For example, if you need to assert strength against an enemy, your heart chakra might willingly give some of it energy to your core chakra so that in that particular scenario, you have less compassion and more strength. Thus, the state of chakras shift and change according to whatever you are dealing with in the moment. While they have general tendencies and traits, nothing in them is ever constant except that they are constantly adjusting.

Chakra Balance - "Just Right"

A balanced chakra does not maintain a centered state at all times, but rather can adjust and manipulate itself to the circumstances and external forces put upon it. Commonly, the state of chakras are described as open or closed. Healers are taught to "open" the chakras. From a very general perception this description is accurate, but upon closer inspection, open and closed is somewhat deceptive because a closed chakra would imply a complete blockage of the energy, which is indication of death. If there is a kink in the hose, the water doesn't flow. If there is a short in the wire, the electricity doesn't conduct and the device does not work. If there is a blockage of an artery of the heart, a heart attack occurs and could be fatal. Thus, healers are not trying to open chakras that are closed, but rather to facilitate optimal flow of the energy that is there. In some cases, turning down the intensity of the energy that is too open facilitates healing, whereas in other cases, turning up the intensity of the energy that is too closed may facilitate healing.

Rather than looking at chakras as open or closed, a better way to describe the state of chakras is to look at them as balanced or excessive or deficient. A Balanced Chakra is when the chakra is able to take in and let go of energy appropriately and is able to adjust to conditions adequately. Like Goldilocks looking for just the right temperature of porridge, the chakras are constantly seeking the just right state in all their characteristics. For example, think of a chakra like the aperture of a camera with many different features to control. In one case, a chakra may be too open, letting in too much energy. Like a camera with the lens too open, it produces a picture that is too light. On the other hand, a chakra may be too closed, not allowing enough energy inside. Like a camera with the lens too closed, it produces a picture that is too dark. In both cases, the picture is difficult to see. However, a chakra isn't just about being open or closed, but about size, and shape, and color, and density, and so forth. Therefore, each of the qualities and characteristics of the chakras is seeking the just right state in any number of various situations. A healthy chakra is one that can adapt and adjust to find balance in any number of circumstances and situations, just like the healthy human body is able to adapt and adjust to the conditions in which it lives.

An ideal balance for one person is not necessarily the same for another person as balance is also determined by genetic coding, environmental conditions, and chakra development. A balanced chakra doesn't depend upon one characteristic alone either. A very large chakra may exhibit imbalances because it is also significantly light and airy, or a tiny chakra that is very dim may exhibit imbalances because it is also extremely dense and heavy. Thus, the balance of your chakras is very individual and particular based upon your lifestyle, your genetics, your development, and your experiences.

Aspects of Each Chakra

The science of diagnosing the specific energetic state of chakras is an intricate and complex science. This book will cover some of the basics by explaining the following for each of the seven main chakras:

> Name & Color
> Governing Realm
> Body Location
> Development Stage
> Ecological Element
> Emotional Balance
> Characteristics of Imbalance
> Balancing Practices & Prescriptions

Name & Color

The word *chakra* is Sanskrit for "wheel" or "disc" as symbolized by the sun, the moon, the earth, the cycle of life, the medicine wheels of ancient cultures, and so much more. The energy of the *chakra* is not just circular in shape, but symbolic of no beginning and no end, the cyclical nature of all things in life.

The Sanskrit Language is a sacred tongue that holds meaning far beyond the literal translations of its words. The sound and vibrations that occur when speaking the words actually serve to tune and adjust the vibrations of the chakras and subtle energies in your body. To understand the symbolism and etymology of the Sanskrit names for the chakras and the vibrational pattern they encode into your system is to have a deeper understanding of how the chakra functions within the whole of your being.

The table below lists the chakra and its Sanskrit name and translation.

Sanskrit Definitions			
Chakra	**Color**	**Sanskrit**	**Translation**
Root	Red	Muladhara	Root Support
Sacral	Orange	Svadhisthana	Sweet Place
Core	Yellow	Manipura	Precious Gem
Heart	Green	Anahata	Not Separate, Unbroken
Throat	Blue	Vissudha	Honest Purity
Third Eye	Indigo	Ajna	Authority, Command
Crown	Violet	Sahasrara	Together with the Whole

Governing Realm

Each chakra serves as the energetic center that governs a different aspect of your life. The body parts, development stages, ecological elements, emotional balance, and other characteristics of the charkas are all symbolic of the governing realm of that chakra.

Governing Realm	
Chakra	**Realm**
Root	Support
Sacral	Joy
Core	Power
Heart	Relationships
Throat	Communication
Third Eye	Insight
Crown	Spirituality

Development Stage

Just as babies are born with all their muscles, but those muscles develop and learn coordination over time, we are born with all our chakras, which also develop and learn coordination over time. While we go through stages of development in our muscular coordination and mental capacity, we also go through similar stages of development in our chakras. The seven major chakras develop incrementally in general coordination with child development stages as highlighted in the list below. Major tragedies, trauma, triumphs, or joys that occur during these various stages of development can directly impact the tendencies and characteristics of the corresponding chakra.The ages listed are approximate and vary for each individual, just as physical and emotional maturity varies.

Chakra Development Stages

Chakra	Development Stage	Development Age
Root	Infancy	Conception – 12 mos
Sacral	Toddler	12mo – 3yrs
Core	Early School	3yrs – 5yrs
Heart	Grade School	6yrs – 9yrs
Throat	Preteen	10yrs – 13yrs
Third Eye	Teenage	14yrs – 18yrs
Crown	Young Adult	19+yrs

Body Location

The seven major chakras are located along the spine, from the base to the crown. The body parts physically located closest to the chakra are directly impacted by the energy and state of the chakra. Injuries, illnesses, or ailments in the body are usually indications of imbalance within the chakra directly connected to that body part.

Body Location	
Chakra	**Body Location**
Root	Feet & Legs
Sacral	Hips & Pelvis
Core	Torso & Abdomen
Heart	Chest & Arms
Throat	Neck & Jaw
Third Eye	Face & Head
Crown	Skull & Brain

Ecological Element

Element	
Chakra	**Natural Element**
Root	Earth
Sacral	Water
Core	Fire
Heart	Air
Throat	Mineral
Third Eye	Nature
Crown	Spirit

Each chakra is symbolic of a natural element. Together the elements of the chakras work together to create an energetic ecosystem which functions best when each of the elements is in balance with the others. Just as a plant needs just the right combination of soil, sun, water, and air, so does your body. You need earth to keep you grounded, water to keep you fluid, sun to give you energy and strength, air to provide space, mineral to give you structure, nature to grow, and spirit to activate your faith. Just as the world goes through cycles of rain and drought, feast and famine, clouds and sun, and so forth, so does your body.

The elements of the chakras mutually support each other. Think of yourself energetically as a tree. You need earth in which to dig your roots and from which to draw up nourishment. You need water and sun to help you grow. At the same time, you provide a home and food for other living beings. As in ecology, the elements go through cycles and phases in accordance with the environment, as do the energies and elements of your chakras.

The elements can also counter-balance each other. For example, too much fire in your core chakra may dry up the water of your sacral chakra, or too much mineral of your throat chakra may starve out the nature of your third eye chakra. At times when your root chakra is imbalanced, it is like the soil for a plant being too dense or too loose. At times when your sacral chakra is imbalanced, it is like a plant being over or under-watered. If a plant is over-watered, it is likely that its soil is rather loose.

Emotional Balance

While generally, a chakra is seeking balance of all its qualities and traits, from density to volume to hue to brightness etc., it is also seeking balance between the individual chakra light emotion and chakra shadow emotion. Each of the seven major chakras of the system govern a different aspect of life, just like each organ of your body manages its own functions within the body. Those aspects of our lives have two sides, a light and a shadow, like the heads and tails of a coin, the yin and the yang.

Emotional Balance		
Chakra	**Light Emotion**	**Shadow Emotion**
Root	Support	Fear
Sacral	Joy	Guilt
Core	Power	Shame
Heart	Love	Grief
Throat	Expression	Repression
Third Eye	Intuition	Illusion
Crown	Faith	Reason

While at first glance, the light of the chakra may appear to be something good, something we want to foster in our lives, and the shadow may appear as something bad, something we want to avoid in our lives. Let's take a step away from the good and bad connotations and apply the language of positive and negative, like positive and negative in electricity, to power and shadow. In order for a battery to work in an electronic device, the positive and negative poles of the battery must line up appropriately and

34

balance each other. Instead of thinking of the light as good and the shadow as bad, think of them as positive and negative ends of a battery, and that you need both. We live in a dualistic world that is filled the a balance of equals and opposites: light/dark, day/night, open/closed, awake/asleep, heavy/light, light/dense, work/play, and so forth. In each of these examples of opposites, a balance between the two is a natural law in our universe.

Let's analyze the root chakra balance of support and fear as an example. While yes, you want to foster support in your life, you also need an appropriate level of fear. Fear is the emotion and energy in your life that protects you, that keeps you safe. If you were to eliminate fear entirely (like shutting off the negative pole of the battery terminal) you might run the risk of running of a cliff because it looks like fun, or touching the hot stove because it looks pretty. Fear is the energy that warns you against things in life that are not safe and supportive. If you have too much support and not enough fear, you might be ungrounded and living in a constant state of risk and danger. If you have too much fear and not enough support, you might be stuck and stagnant in your life, unable to move. You need both to complement each other, to balance each other.

Characteristics of Imbalance

A **Deficient Chakra** is one that is lacking in its Light energy, and thus excessive in its Shadow energy, like a ligh bulb that is too dim, or a water faucet without enough pressure, or a stereo with the volume too low. A deficient chakra often means that it compensates with excessive Shadow. As an example, someone with not enough pleasure (sacral chakra) in life often lives with an excess of guilt.

An **Excessive Chakra** is one that holds too much Light energy, like a refrigerator that runs constantly or a computer tower that runs too hot. For example, an excessive core chakra is like a plant that has too much sun exposure and its leaves are dry and brittle.

An excessive chakra often means that it compensates with excessive Light. As an example, someone who exhibits a huge ego of power (core chakra) has very little shame and tends to bully others.

The **Extreme Chakra** is one that fluctuates from excessive to deficient, often depending upon the circumstance or situation at hand. This chakra may appear balanced, but rather, it swings from one end of the spectrum to the other, living on the extremes, feast or famine, drought or flood. The shifts may occur based upon certain circumstances in life, or it may fluctuate based on the other environmental factors such as people you encounter. For example, someone who is extremely talkative while with family and close friends may also be extremely shy and nonverbal when with strangers is an example of an extreme throat chakra. It is as if this person has a control valve on the chakra that only has two settings, strong or weak. Like a water tap that either barely drips or gushes uncontrollably.

The **Dominant Chakra** is one that indicates a particular inherent gift or talent. A dominant chakra does not mean that it is always in balance, but rather that it is a specific talent. This is the chakra that is least likely to go out of balance. However, if it does go out of balance, it results in the most dramatic effects. The governing traits of one's dominant chakra are skills and traits that come naturally to that individual. For example, a dominant core chakra is someone who naturally feels self-empowered, has a healthy self-esteem, and has a good moral compass that turns on just enough shame to stop him from behaving outside what is true to his own personal power. Such a person often becomes someone who helps others feel empowered, or provides strength and power for those who are weakened by circumstances or challenges. If you find a career or life venture that is in line with your dominant chakra, typically your life is easier and your chakras stay more balanced.

Life Lesson

When an individual chakra is balanced, you are experiencing a state of peace and content within the realm of your life that chakra governs. If the chakra is imbalanced, you are experiencing opportunities in your life to learn and grow. The list below offers simple phrases to describe the lessons you can learn by tuning and adjusting the imbalances in each chakra.

Life Lessons	
Chakra	**Life Lesson**
Root	Stand Your Ground
Sacral	Go with the Flow
Core	Access Your Strength
Heart	Give and Receive
Throat	Speak Your Truth
Third Eye	Focus Your Vision
Crown	Live with Awareness

Balancing Practices & Prescriptions

Energy is neither created nor destroyed. It simply moves around and changes forms. It can be concentrated or diffused. Unlike the physical muscles of your body that need to be built and conditioned over time, the energy in chakras and that flows through your nadis can be accessed immediately by knowing how to tune the chakras to move the energy most efficiently throughout the body. Thus, healing from the energetic level can be accessed almost immediately by tuning and balancing the chakras. Such medicine has been provided in all cultures since the beginning of time. Chinese and Ayurvedic medicine work on both the physical and energetic levels, as does the practices of yoga and shamanic rituals. Practices such as Healing Touch, Reiki, QiGong, and others, as energetic healing are increasing in popularity across the globe. These practices all require a trained practitioner to provide the healing and, like seeing a western medicine doctor, can be costly and time consuming. In addition, when you see these practitioners, your chakras are usually borrowing energy from the practitioner, but maintaining that energy for yourself outside the care of the practitioner is challenging. This is why you may feel much better while in their immediate care of a practitioner; however, over time the chakras do revert to their prior tendencies, which is why the effects of energy healing and bodywork isn't always long-lasting. The challenge is keeping your chakras balanced or developing the ability to adjust them appropriately. Thus, just like the muscles of your body, your chakras need exercising and conditioning to maintain optimal energy flow.

You can provide yourself with simple forms of energetic medication to balance the chakras through practices such as: body alignment, exercise, diet, interaction with the nature, and more. In fact, as you read through the rest of this book, you may find that you naturally gravitate toward energetic medicine for imbalances without even knowing it. The key to optimal health is both awareness of your body and energy and a consistent practice. Just as a consistent healthy diet and exercise regiment helps promote optimal physical health, a consistent healthy awareness and energy practice help promote optimal chakra balance.

This book is not meant to replace western medicine, but as a means to supplement it. In many cases, such as bacterial infections, broken bones, or the need for surgical procedures, chakra ailment requires traditional medicine to facilitate the healing process. Chakra balancing supports healing.

The practices and prescriptions in this book are practical and relatively easy to fulfill in your average everyday life. They are not likely to have dramatic side effects, but can offer great benefits. In these types of prescriptions, the more often you can infuse them into your everyday life, the more benefits you will see. A consistent practice provides the most optimal benefits on all levels: physically, spiritually, energetically, psychologically, and mentally. You will find that your chakras have tendencies to slip in and out of balance based on several factors in your life, but you can counter these effects by applying a consistent and dedicated practice.

However, as with anything, moderation is always the best policy. Like western medicine, higher dosages of energetic medicine such as deep spiritual ritual may have unexpected side effects. If you think you need higher doses of energetic medicine, consult with a practitioner skilled and trained in that form of energetic medicine to provide the service to you.

Just Right Doesn't Mean There is a Wrong

"There is no right or wrong, only right or left."
~African Proverb

A balanced chakra is no more right than an extreme or deficient or excessive chakra. In fact, at some point in time, we have all experienced deficient, excessive, extreme, and balanced chakras. This is the human condition. To live and experience too much and not enough and go back and forth is all part of the process of what makes the stories of our lives interesting. If Goldilocks didn't have different porridges and chairs and beds to try out, there wouldn't have been a story in the first place. The hard bed was perfect for Papa Bear, while the cold porridge was exactly how Mama Bear liked it. The goal is not to achieve and maintain balance all the time. The Snow White story shows that external forces have an impact on the chakras and throw them out of balance all the time. The goal is to be adaptable and be able to adjust your energies according to those external forces. The goal is also not to make your chakras look and move and behave like those of others. While each of the seven dwarves was similar, the popular Disney movie showed that each dwarf has his or her own personality, traits, gifts, talents, and short-comings. Life is simply about experiencing all levels and playing the game of finding what works for you in that moment of time. Both Goldilocks and Snow White learned listen to themselves. The goal is to adjust for you what is just right in any given moment.

CHAPTER 4

The Root Chakra

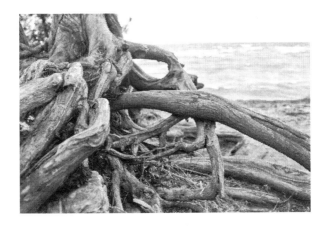

Sanskrit - Muladhara

Mula = Root Network
Dhara = Support or Foundation

Definition

The color of the root chakra is red, like deep soil. The root chakra is a reticulated root system of your body, used to draw energetic nourishment from Mother Earth, providing support, foundation, stability, and safety.

Governing Realm - Support

Home
Health
Family
Safety
Support
Finances

The power of the root chakra is Support, governing home, health, family, nourishment, survival, and other basic needs. A balanced root chakra supports a solid home, a supportive family, a healthy body, a financially secure job, and good nourishing food on your table. Somewhere in history the honor and credence that is due to Mother Earth (ecology) as our support system was shifted to money (economics). Ironically, the prefix "eco-" relates to environment (earth), and the suffix "-nomics "relates to 'law'. Thus, economics literally translates to 'law of the environment'.

The energetic nourishment of life comes from a support system of people and things that live and work together, mutually supporting each other, like an ecosystem. In an ecosystem, you tend the garden, cultivate the soil, water the plants, providing your love and labor, and eventually you are provided with fruit that nourishes you in return. Your root chakra governs your ability to support yourself within the context of your environment.

Body Location - Feet & Legs

The body parts connected to the Root Chakra are the Legs and Feet, including toes, heels, ankles, knees, thighs and calves, everything from the hinges of your hips down to the tips of your toes. This includes your low back as that is base, or root, of your spine. If you have issues with any of these body parts, chances are, you are also struggling in your life in one of the following areas: home, family, health, support, finances, and safety. Energetically, Mother Earth provides all of these things to you through your root chakra.

This little piggy went to the market.

This little piggy stayed home.

This little piggy ate roast beef.

This little piggy had none.

And this little piggy went wee wee wee all the way home.

The favorite nursery rhyme "This Little Piggy" combined with wiggling each of the five toes of your foot is symbolic of the energies of the root chakra as they are connected to the toes. A balanced root chakra means that you are grounded and rooted, but free to explore the world around you as well. Thus, like the piggies, part of your foot stays rooted in home while another goes away to the market. One of the piggies takes in food while another doesn't, representing balance. Perhaps the baby piggy is the most symbolic as it cries all the way home. Is that cry a cry of joy or a cry of fear? Perhaps it is meant to be ambiguous as a means of showing that the experience of life is a balance of joy and fear.

While your feet are what support you on the ground, your legs are what you use to move around. A balanced root chakra is both rooted to the earth and free to navigate through experiences of life. If you suffer from injuries or pains in your legs, chances are that you are also experiencing the inability to stay rooted and/or move and navigate the experiences of your life. These symptoms typically manifest in the areas of your life that surround your home, family, basic needs, health, and support.

As an example, your low back is the part of your body that supports the largest mass of the weight of your body. When you have more to support in your life, both physically and energetically, your low back is going to feel the weight. In today's modern world, financial worries are symptomatic of feeling unsupported in life, which often manifests in low back pain.

Your feet and legs represent your ability to stand your ground in your life. If you have difficulty standing on your own feet, it could be because you have imbalances in your root chakra.

Development Stage - Infant

The Root Chakra develops from the time of conception through infancy. What was happening with your family and home during the time your mother was pregnant with you and throughout your infancy? To gain a better understanding of the development of your root chakra, take some time to reflect and research the following during the time of your mother's pregnancy and your infancy:

- The physical health of yourself and your immediate family, particularly your mother
- Your home
- Your emotional support system, especially from your immediate and extended family
- Your parents' financial circumstances
- Whether or not your were breast-fed

If any of the above factors are challenged during the mother's pregnancy and the baby's infancy, the root chakra could have difficulty developing. The resulting imbalance could manifest as scarcity or overabundance. For example, an infant who is not adequately supported through infancy, and lives in a family who struggles with major health issues, financial strain, lack of emotional support, and real or perceived homelessness may struggle with those same issues throughout his life. On the other hand, an infant who is overly nurtured and over-protected may become dependent on others to provide for him and never build the ability to take care of his own financial and supporting needs in life. In both cases, these individuals may grow into adults who have difficulty providing for their own basic needs because their root chakra development was stunted during infancy.

This is not to say that someone cannot adequately compensate for inadequacies that developed during infancy, just that development was challenged. Individuals with root chakra imbalances may build their root chakra muscles over time and learn to compensate for that which was not provided in their infancy.

Health

When women get pregnant, they are likely to take extra precautions to maintain a healthy lifestyle because their own health will directly impact the health of their babies. If members of your family, particularly your mother, struggle with significant health challenges, particularly during the time of pregnancy and infancy, your root chakra will be affected.

Home

While some conditions are inherent, other circumstances are environmental - nature vs. nurture. As your home is the environment in which you live and spend most of your time, the status of your home affects your root chakra. Infants in particular spend most of their time at home. Thus, if the home is challenged or unstable during infancy, it can impact the development of the root chakra. A common phenomenon for pregnant mother's is that they go through a heavy 'nesting' phase in which they prepare the home for the arrival of the baby. The more nurturing and supportive the home, the healthier the baby's root chakra develops.

Emotional Support

An infant's main concern in life is basic needs, such as food and shelter. Babies cry when they are hungry, cold, or just want a cuddle. The cuddling serves as emotional support for a soul new to this world. This emotional support comes most directly from the immediate family, particularly the mother and father. If the mother and father feel supported themselves by their own family and friends, they are likely able to provide emotional support for their infant. The broader the emotional support system in the function of family, extended family, and friends, the more supported the baby feels. This is the concept of the adage "it takes a village to raise a child" at work. The more supportive the family's community, particularly family, the more supported the baby feels.

Finances

In modern culture, our homes, our food, and our access to healthcare are all supported by money, economics. Money is necessary to buy all the basic needs that support your root chakra. We need money to pay rent or mortgages for our homes. We need money to buy food for our tables. We need money to buy clothes and blankets. We need money to pay our doctors. Thus, your relationship with money directly impacts your root chakra. Without enough money, we live in fear of not having our basic needs met as we cannot pay the bills for our homes or purchase food for our tables. If the family is financially secure at the time we are infants and our basic needs are easily met through financial means, we are likely to have a more solid root chakra development. If the family is struggling to buy baby clothes, or the home is threatened during infancy, it will impact the ability of the root chakra to develop.

Breast-Feeding

Early breast milk is considered liquid gold to newborns because it provides rich nutrients and antibodies to nourish and protect the baby. Within a few days the breast milk matures to provide just the right combination of fat, sugar, water, and protein to help the baby grow. Breast-milk is easy to digest, supporting digestive functioning, providing the perfect nutrition in just the right quantity for the growing baby. Breast milk provides hormones and antibodies to support immune functioning and prevent and heal from disease. The bonding between mother and baby during breastfeeding provides valuable psychological and sociological benefits to support a sense of security, safety, and prevention of fear of abandonment.

Ecological Element - Earth

The element for the root chakra is EARTH, symbolizing the Divine Mother who provides support, nourishment, home, comfort, and unconditional love. Mother Earth loves all living beings equally. She provides a home and support for the criminal as well as the righteous, the honest and the dishonest, the virtuous and the wretched. She is the grandmother who wants everyone to feel at home, nourished, loved, respected, and supported. Mother Earth gives, and she gives abundantly. All creatures are her children, and she allows them all to walk on her and reap from her abundance equally. The gravitational pull of earth ensures that Mother Earth never kicks anyone out of her home.

While Mother Earth never says no, she cannot force her abundance on anyone anymore than a mother can force a baby to breast-feed. Thus, to balance the root chakra is to develop a relationship with Mother Earth, to latch, like a baby latches to the Mother's breast, and receive an abundance of comfort, support, stability, foundation, home, and love.

The Tree of Life: As Above, So Below

Perhaps the best analogy to understand the element of Earth is to compare your body to a tree. Trees have a complex root system that digs into the soil of earth both to provide foundation and stability, and also to draw up nourishment.

Many religious and spiritual traditions hold the Tree of Life as a mystical concept of the inter-connectedness of all life on earth. The Tree of Life has as many branches into the sky as it has roots

"As above, so below" is applied in the simple law of physics "the force of any action creates an equal and opposite reaction." In other words, "what goes up must come down" is reversed to "that which pushes downwards must reverberate upwards." The roots and branches of a tree are only one example of this universal law of life. Other examples include the action of a yo-yo or the bouncing of a super ball on the ground. The force you exert on the ball or yo-yo pushing down is reverberated upwards. Applying this concept to your body and your root chakra means that as you root into Mother Earth, you grow and branch out into the world.

Ashes to Ashes – Dust to Dust

In many traditions, from Africa to China, Egyptian to Mayan, Christian to Islam, man is said to have been made from the mud, dust, or clay of the earth. When we die, the body is returned to the earth in burial or scattered as ashes.

> *"Lord God formed man of dust from the ground, and breathed in his nostrils the breath of life; and man became a living being." (Genesis 2:7)*

> *"You shall eat the plants of the field. In the sweat of your face you shall eat bread till you return to the ground, for out of it you were taken; you are dust, and to dust you shall return." (Genesis 3:18-19)*

Symbolically and spiritually, man is made from the dust of earth, grows from the soil of earth and is returned at death as ashes to the bed of earth. The element of Earth provides all the nourishment of basic needs. Mother Earth is our home. She provides food for our nourishment, and holds us unconditionally to her. Since we are made from her, we also hold within us all the qualities and traits of Mother Earth.

Biologically, our bodies are made up of the same basic molecules and elements of the earth, just configured in different formations and densities. Just as we feed off the plants and animals that roam the earth, once our bodies are committed to the ground after death, they decompose and serve as nourishment to the creatures and critters of the earth and provide fertilizer to the plants that grow from that soil. The whole process is cyclical, just as the process of being born of dust and returning to dust is one large cycle. The concept of the cycle is that all things return from whence they came, mutually supporting one another as a piece of the whole.

When we function as a piece of the whole, we recognize the interconnectedness and mutual support of the cycles of the universe. However, when we struggle with issues of not being supported in the basic needs of our lives such as home, food, family, health, or finances, we need to connect with the energy of Mother Earth. Imbalances in Earth energy in your system result in issues of scarcity in life. Balanced earth results in a feeling of support and an ability to provide support to others, abundance.

Emotional Balance - Support/Fear

A healthy and balanced root chakra manifests in a healthy relationship with support and fear in your life.

The light emotion of the root chakra is support. Support is the feeling that all your needs are met, that you are adequately supported to survive the situation at hand. When you feel too supported in your life you may be consistently ignoring warnings of danger in the form of fear.

The shadow emotion of the root chakra is fear. When we are in danger, or we suffer a loss of a loved one, or we face a significant health challenge, or we endure the relocation of our home, or we face unemployment or change in jobs, a certain level of fear of the unknown is a healthy way to keep us cautious and safe. Excessive concern over physical health, home, family, finances, employment, or food usually is the result of an unhealthy level of fear, which is indication of an imbalance of the root chakra.

When your root chakra is balanced, you feel safe and supported in all that you do while also able to recognize when safety and support is not available and to either avoid that situation or to find the support necessary before engaging in the situation.

Characteristics of Imbalance

Excessive Root Chakra

An excessive root chakra means too much focus in life is put upon creating, maintaining, and protecting support in your life, usually out of fear of not being supported. Symptoms may include:

- swelling of the legs and feet
- tumors (particularly in the lower body)
- low back pain
- overweight or obesity
- over-eating
- hoarding
- resistance to relocation or travel
- stagnancy
- preoccupation with safety & security
- paranoia & excessive or irrational fear
- extreme focus on the home
- penny-pinching
- anxiety
- stubbornness

On an average day of channel flipping, one can see many examples of excessive root chakra in weight loss infomercials, hoarding reality shows, emergency room dramas, murder mysteries, and depictions of dangerous careers. A great metaphor

Deficient Root Chakra

A deficient root chakra means not enough focus in life is put upon creating, maintaining, and protecting the concept of support and safety in your life. Symptoms may include:

- anorexia

- underweight

- brittle bones

- homelessness

- feeling of not-belonging

- excessive relocation and/or travel

- debt

- inability to keep a job or home

- inability to commit

- neediness

- tendency to give away or lose things

- forgetting to eat or tendency to skip meals

- excessive risk-taking

Those commercials calling for donations to support various charities to feed the hungry depicting pictures of hungry children with bloated bellies or images of homeless people begging for food on the streets are examples of deficient root chakra imbalances. A great metaphor to describe someone with an deficient root chakra is to think of them as a tree or plant whose roots are so shallow that even the slightest wind or rain would blow or wash it away.

Extreme Root Chakra

An extreme root chakra means that energy shifts from too much focus on basic needs to complete disregard of needs and support. A great metaphor to describe the extreme root chakra is the concept of "feast or famine." As an example, in an effort to maintain balance, someone with an extreme root chakra may struggle to meet basic needs for a time, and then flood themselves with extravagances when given the opportunity. Symptoms may include:

- bulimia

- hoarding in some areas of life while neediness in others

- all or nothing attitude

- overly cautious and extremely risky

The extreme chakra is difficult to diagnose, and even more difficult to balance, especially because on some level, the chakra finds its own state of balance by swinging from one state to the extreme opposite. Often, the extreme chakra is a result of a conflict of nature vs. nurture. For example, you may inherit a deficient root chakra from your mother, but her efforts to compensate resulted in over-protectiveness creating an excessive root chakra. Your energy gets confused by this battle and finds balance by swinging from one extreme to the other.

Root Chakra Dominance

A dominant root chakra means that you have particular skill and talent in the areas of support, home, family, foundation, money, and health. These individuals have an innate ability to make sure basic needs are met. People who have a dominant root chakra are exceptional at making others feel at home in any situation. They may do this by providing nourishing food, welcoming people into their homes, caring for the sick, loaning money, or making people feel like they are part of the family.

Careers that are root chakra dominant include:

- farmers & gardeners

- home-makers

- home-builders

- realtors

- chefs & cooks

- doctors

- social workers

- money managers

- bankers

- police officers

Life Lesson - Stand Your Ground

The Donkey in the Well

There was a farmer who owned many farm animals. One day, one of his donkeys fell into a dry well. The farmer tried to get the animal out for a long time but all his efforts were fruitless. Finally, the farmer decided it was probably impossible to get it out and also, the animal was old and the well was dry anyway, so it just wasn't worth it to try and retrieve the donkey. So, the farmer asked his neighbors to come over and help him cover up the well. They all grabbed shovels and began to shovel dirt and sand into the well. After a few shovel loads, the farmer looked down into the well to see what was happening and was astonished at what he saw - With every shovel of dirt that hit its back, the donkey was shaking it off and taking a step up. Pretty soon, to everyone's amazement, the donkey stepped up over the edge of the well and trotted off.

Moral: Whenever you get challenged, shake it off and step up. The ground is always underneath you.

In the beginning of this story, both the donkey and the farmer are afraid that the donkey will meet his final demise. In the end, the donkey had two choices, to succumb to death by burial in the deep well, or to shake off the dirt of each shovelful and step up, as he ultimately did, to his own salvation.

When you are challenged in your life by root chakra imbalances, the lessons surround fear and support. While the donkey did depend upon others, the farmer, for his support, the farmer could not have saved the donkey if he didn't want to be saved and participate in the process himself. The same is the case for most issues of root chakra imbalance. While you may need to support of others to take care of you, on some level, you must face your fear and participate in your own healing. You must learn to stand on the ground underneath you and support yourself because ultimately, no one else can take care of your needs completely. It's like the old adage "you can lead a horse to water, but you cannot force it to drink." Others can care for you, but that care only goes so far. Ultimately, you must always stand on your own two feet and support and care for yourself.

Balancing Practices & Prescriptions

Diet & Nutrition

A **deficient root chakra** is lacking in density, thus eating foods with more density and that provide density will help nourish the energy of the root chakra. Root vegetables such as potatoes, yams, onions, carrots, turnips, and other foods that grow directly in the soil are extremely healing to the deficient root chakra because they bring the energy of the soil directly into your system, reminding you that Mother Earth is your home and support, both inside and outside your body. The deep red color of foods like beets and red meat is the same color as the root chakra, bringing that vibration and energy to your system. In addition, red meats and nuts are rich in protein that provides density and sustenance to your system. Whole grains such as brown rice, couscous, quinoa, millet, and barley break down to provide fuel for your muscles. As with all foods, take these foods in moderation to avoid swinging from deficiency into excessiveness or extreme imbalances. In addition, often a deficient root chakra may be a result of hunger. Eating is a very grounding activity that can provide energy to a light and deficient root chakra. If you feel light-headed, spacey, airy, ungrounded, or flighty, eating a good meal can be simple fix.

An **excessive root chakra** has too much density, so foods that are watery and airy can help to lighten the density. Fruits and vegetables, particularly those that leave a puddle on your cutting board or those that have large spaces of air when you cut inside them help to loosen the soil of a dense root chakra. Eating more vegetables that grow on vines and fruits that grow on trees can help connect you with air and water. These may include peppers, tomatoes, apples, citrus fruit, berries, cucumbers, and zucchini.

The **extreme root chakra** swings from over-dense to over-light depending upon the circumstance or situation, so balance and equilibrium is vital. The best diet for the extreme root chakra is one that provides an even balance of both dense and light foods. Instead of a meal of meat and potatoes, consider meat and peppers. Other foods that are supportive of balancing the extreme root chakra are those that grow on the ground but also have elements of water and air within them, such as ... that grow on the soil but are juicy and airy on the inside.

Body Mechanics - Root Embrace

Solid positioning of your legs and feet establishes a safe foundation and thus provides healing energy of safety, foundation, support, structure, and stability, all the powers of the root chakra. This action will add energy to the deficient root chakra, extract energy from the excessive root chakra, bring equilibrium to the extreme chakra, and support maintenance of the balanced root chakra. The simple action of consciously "latching" your feet to the earth and engaging your inner thigh muscles provides just the right combination of stability and structure to align any position.

Think of the arches of your feet as the lips that pucker on the breast of Mother Earth. If you look at the anatomy of the foot, it is shaped somewhat like a half suction cup. When you place your foot consciously and evenly distribute the weight of your foot, your foot creates a sort of puckering effect on the floor. Then, the puckering is channeled through your legs, like straws, to your torso. This effect is created physically in the body through activation of the adductor muscles of your inner thighs, which are used primarily to bring your legs in toward your body. Since the effect you are trying to create is to bring energy and nourishment from Mother Earth into your body, you want to use the muscles that ADD (adductors) to your system.

Since your feet are the lips that energetically latch to the breast of Mother Earth, the "latch" of your feet to the nipple of Mother Earth is vital. One way to ensure a good latch of your body to Mother Earth is to consciously place your feet, evenly distributing your weight.

When standing unconsciously, it is common to shift your weight from one foot to the other as a means of sharing the burden of holding up your body. When you depend on one part of your foot to hold the majority of your weight, after a short time, the muscles required to support your weight will fatigue, so you shift your weight to a different position to apply the majority of the weight to a different group of muscles.

If you latch your feet to the earth and evenly distribute the weight across all the muscles of your feet and legs, the alignment of your body provides support through the architecture of your bones, allowing your muscles to share the burden and last longer.

To do this, stand with your feet hip width apart (about 6-8 inches). Look down and turn your heels out slightly so that your feet are actually straight. For many people, this will feel slightly pigeon-toed, but when you look, your feet should be straight. If you were to draw a line around the edges of your feet, it would form a rectangle, not a trapezoid. Aligning your heels straight causes your feet to engage more solidly with the floor. In addition, this slight rotation of your heels sets the ball of your thigh bone (femur) into the hip socket more securely, creating a stronger and more stable connection between your hip and your leg and your foot. By turning your feet straight, your sit bones will separate slightly, allowing the femur bone easier access to the socket, and thus the bones of your legs and hips plug together more squarely and solidly, creating a solid foundation.

This is not to say that you should stand upright and evenly on two feet at all times. Just as an infant does not spend the entire day suckling at the mother's breast, you do not need to spend the entire day latching to Mother Earth through your feet and legs. However, when you feel like you need a little nurturing, nourishment, support, or foundation, the simple act of consciously aligning your feet to properly "latch" to Mother Earth several times a day will support the balance and development of the root chakra energy in your system.

Your adductor muscles are located on your inner thighs, and are quite possibly the most under-appreciated muscles of your legs. These muscles symbolize the action of "adding in" energy. Think of these muscles as little straws, or ducts, that suck in energy to your system. They AD-DUCT.

An easy way to learn how to engage these muscles is to stand with your feet even and place a four-inch yoga block between your thighs. The slight hugging of the block between your thighs engages your adductor muscles causing a slight internal rotation of your upper thigh that creates a spiraling suction sensation from the arches of your feet right up your legs into your torso.

This action creates both a rooting sensation down through your feet and a lifting sensation up your legs. Scientifically, this action is the universal law of physics "the force of any action creates an equal and opposite reaction." Thus, pushing down in your feet creates an equal and opposite lifting sensation in your upper body. Many people report feelings of becoming more stable, balanced, rooted, plugged into the ground as well as lighter, freer, and more lifted.

You can do many little things throughout your day to remind your body of the support in your world and to connect with Mother's nourishment through your feet and legs.

- Hug a yoga block between your thighs while doing dishes, cooking, brushing your teeth, standing in line, or any other mundane home task that requires standing.

- Watch your feet as you take short walks, particularly on the beach or in the snow where you can see your footprints to assess your heel alignment. Make an effort to place each step with feet parallel rather than slightly duck-footed (toes out) or pigeon-toed (toes in).

- To relieve low back tension, sit up tall and root both feet into the ground. Activate your adductor muscles by squeezing your two fists between your knees.

Breathing Practice - Belly Breath

Breath provides almost eighty percent of the energy you need to get through your day, while food provides only about twenty percent. Thus, when you are feeling energetically undernourished, a good deep breath can provide the support and sustenance you may need. In addition, increasing your breath capacity to breathe deep into the lower lungs has a very grounding effect. More often than not, average everyday breathing is conducted mainly in the upper chest, shallow. A deep breath into the lower lungs is like taking a big drink of nourishment. To do this, place your hands on your belly and exhale all your air. As you inhale, breathe first into your upper chest, then your ribs, and finally your belly, allowing your belly to expand. Then, as you exhale, breathe out first from your belly, then your ribs, and finally your upper chest. This is called three-part breath as you visualize the path of the air through throat down your lungs and eventually extending your belly and back again.

58

Exercise

When you are lacking support and foundation in a **deficient root chakra**, restorative yoga is a very gentle form of exercise where you lay on bolsters, blankets and other props that provide full support and foundation. You will open your body while being fully supported by the energy of Mother Earth through the floor. Many yoga studios offer restorative classes that are easy and accessible to all body types and fitness levels.

When you are stuck and overburdened by an **excessive root chakra**, taking a simple stroll gets the fluids in your system flowing to break up any stagnancy and density. It is like a good aeration and watering of the lawn of your body.

Elemental Practices - Engaging with Earth

Spending time with earth, in physical contact with the soil of Mother Earth can also be extremely healing to the root chakra imbalances of all types because it is a reminder that Mother Earth provides all, and on a spiritual level, you came from Mother Earth and you will return to her after you die.

Anytime you expose your feet to the world, you are opening the tiny channels of your root chakra more directly to gain access to energy. When you get a pedicure, you are cleaning out tiny pores making a more clear passage for energy to access your system through your feet. When you receive reflexology or foot rubs the nerve endings of your entire body are stimulated at your feet and the energy channels are cleared to receive better flow and nourishment. Walking barefoot on a beach exercises all the muscles, tendons, ligaments, and tissues of your feet and ankles, providing more open channels.

Placing your bare feet directly on Mother Earth is like attaching the lips of your energetic system directly to the source of nourishment. If you feel a particular need for support and love and nourishment in your life due to trauma or tragedy or stress in your family or home, try going for a short walk with bare feet.

Kneeling to the earth and digging your hands into rich soil for gardening is like cleaning the weeds of your life and exposing yourself to the rich nutrient of the soil of your being. In addition, by growing your own food in gardens, you are learning to work in partnership with Mother Earth to provide the needs of your life to yourself.

Mindful Concentration Techniques

The following prescriptions are more spiritually based practices that are balancing and healing for the root chakra.

- Meditating on the color RED
- Offering gratitude to EARTH
- Visualizing your own ROOTS

Journaling Topics

1. Do you have issues with your feet or legs? Do you have body awareness of your internal thigh muscles and the arches of your feet? Do you notice a difference in your support, your stance, your energy when you engage these muscles? How can you apply these simply physical actions to your life? How can you pay better attention to your feet and legs and support the development and use and function of these parts of your body?

2. What is your relationship to your own mother and grandmother? Have you translated your own childhood nurturing from your physical parents to your adult life? How can you appreciate the Divine Mother more in your life? How can you better understand the unconditional love of Mother Earth in your life?

3. What is your relationship to abundance? Are you a giver or a taker? How might you balance the two? Are you open to receive the abundance that is available to you? When someone offers you a gift, do you refuse? If yes, why? Do you find

yourself giving of your time or energy when you would be better of taking care of your own needs first?

4. What is your relationship to money? Do you define abundance as purely economic or financial? Do you allow your financial status to dictate your happiness or sense of success?

CHAPTER 5

The Sacral Chakra

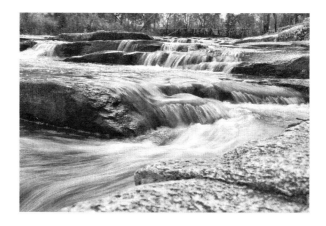

Sanskrit - Svadhisthana

Svad = Pleasant, Sweet
Histhana = One's Own Place

Definition

The svadhisthana, located in the center of your pelvis, is the womb of your being, that pleasurable sweet place of your Self. It is the container of your experiences of life and your ability to taste the sweet nectar of those experiences.

Governing Realm - Pleasure

Play
Recreation
Sexuality
Creativity
Artistry
Fun

The power of the sacral chakra is Pleasure, governing play, joy, sexuality, creativity, artistry, fun, and adventure. A balanced sacral chakra supports a healthy enjoyment of all the experiences and processes of life.

Body Location - Hips & Pelvis

The body part connected to the Sacral Chakra is the pelvis, including hips, reproductive organs, buttocks, and lower digestive tract, everything contained within the pelvic bowl. To become conscious and aware of how you hold your pelvis is to become consciously aware of your ability to be flexible and go with the flow of life.

Think of your pelvis as a bowl that holds the liquid sweetness of your life. As your body is composed mostly of water, you want to keep yourself hydrated, both physically and spiritually. That liquid needs to be both held in the bowl but also churned and cycled through the bowl, just like blood through the heart. If the bowl tilts too much in one direction or another, the liquid gets spilled, leaving your experience of life dry, brittle, rigid, and stiff. If the liquid in the bowl doesn't have an opportunity to move around, it gets stagnant and stale, like a scummy pond. Physiologically, many of your lymph nodes and major arteries are located at your hip joints. These pockets of juice need to be pressed and squeezed to pump the hormones and antibodies of your lymphatic fluids and to churn the blood through your body. Think of these hormones as happy juices and the antibodies as little warriors that fight off illness and negativity.

While pelvic alignment provides for optimal flow of fluid and energy through your system, the curvature of your spine, particularly your lumbar spine, provides the ability to direct the flow. Stability is necessary, but it must not be rigid. It must have a degree of flexibility. Your ability to manipulate your limbs in various directions to do many things comes first from the center column of your spine, which is why it is made up of many little bones stacked together. Each vertebra is independent and can move slightly different from the others. However, when one vertebra is moved, it triggers a domino effect through the whole spine, pushing energy through your body in various ways. This is why the spine is mostly straight (representing stability) but also somewhat curved (representing flexibility).

A healthy spine with an even balance of stability and flexibility provides you with the ability to experience the fullness of life. Like the Sacral Chakra definition, it provides the ability to taste the sweetness of life. Think of your spine as a central river, like the Mississippi River, with various tributaries branching into it. The lumbar spine is like the mouth of the river that meets the ocean. The flow of the liquid of your body follows the flow of gravity, like the flow of the river seeking the ocean. The flow of energy of your body is like the undercurrent of a river that provides its ability to push uphill when necessary. If you can maintain stability from your pelvis, which is connected to the largest vertebrae of your spine, you can learn to more directly control the flow of energy through each vertebra to the rest of your body.

Development Stage - Toddler

The Sacral Chakra develops during the time of toddlerhood, roughly between the ages of twelve to twenty-four months. The balance of your sacral chakra is somewhat connected to what was happening in your life during your toddler years and how you were allowed to express your desire to explore, play, and experience pleasure. By the time children reach toddlerhood, they are developed enough to move around and have a sense of curiosity and adventure. Children at this age are explorers, adventurers, and the world is their playground. To gain a better understanding of the development of your sacral chakra, take some time to reflect and remember the following during the time of your toddlerhood:

- The freedom your parents allowed you to explore your world

- Opportunities provided to you to venture into new territory

- Your accessibility to play and joy

- Your family's tendencies towards joy and play and fun versus work and discipline and responsibility

- Your family's tendencies towards perfectionism and structure versus creativity and adventure

Anal- Retentiveness

Toddlerhood is the time where children go through toilet training. The term "anal-retentiveness" is used in common language to describe a person who is rigid in personality, obsessive in adherence to details. While originally derived from Freud's theory that children who deal with difficulties during toddlerhood develop anal-retentive personalities, theories now state that parental attitudes have a stronger impact on child development. Energetically, both are true. If a child is raised by "anal-retentive" parents who are rigid in discipline and structure, his or her sacral chakra development can be stunted and causing imbalances.

For example, if you were toilet trained on a strict rigid schedule, you were essentially trained to control your fluid systems of your body based on a schedule which limits your body's ability to "go with the flow" of life, but rather restricting you to tight structures and schedules.

Addiction

When you are not allowed or provided with ample opportunities in life to explore and play and seek out pleasure, your life may become overwhelmed with work, structure and discipline. Quite often addiction to mind-altering substances or behaviors that create elevated hormonal releases (alcoholism, drug addiction, sex addiction, exercise addiction) results as a means of seeking pleasure when it cannot otherwise be reached. These behaviors and tendencies are inherent. If you were born to parents with addictive behaviors or tendencies, and particularly if your parent(s) or other care-giving family members succumbed to addictive behaviors in your presence during your toddlerhood (because in toddlerhood your sacral chakra is developing and more susceptible to contagious energies of pleasure), you are more likely to have imbalances in your sacral chakra that may manifest in similar addictive behaviors or tendencies.

Terrible Two's & Guilt

A common phrase to describe the stages of toddlerhood is "the terrible twos" because two and three year olds are so creative and energetic. Toddlers are developing their motor skills in a way that they can move about more freely and thus use their bodies to explore a wider experience of their worlds. This gets them into trouble when they do things like climb bookshelves or insert their fingers in the coils of the back of the refrigerator. Parents spend their days chasing their toddlers around telling them "no" as a means of keeping them safe from potential dangers that the children do not perceive. If "no" is too often coupled with "bad girl" or "bad boy", an unhealthy emotion of guilt may result, and the sacral chakra may develop into imbalance.

If any of the above factors are challenged during the toddlerhood the sacral chakra could have difficulty developing and manifest in issues of imbalance in terms of joy and guilt, pleasure and responsibility, work and play. For example, a toddler who is not allowed appropriate levels of play and adventure and lives in a family who struggles with workaholism and perfectionism may struggle with those same issues throughout his life. On the other hand, a toddler who is given few boundaries and little structure may become dependent on others to provide for him and never build the ability to take responsibility and get work done. In both cases, these individuals may grow into adults who have difficulty balancing work and play in life because their sacral chakras are imbalanced.

This is not to say that one cannot compensate for inadequacies that developed during toddlerhood, just that development was challenged. Individuals with sacral chakra imbalances may build their sacral chakra muscles over time and learn to compensate and live happy balanced lives of work and play.

Ecological Element - Water

The element for the sacral chakra is WATER, symbolic of cleansing, purification, reconciliation, rejuvenation, spirituality, and creativity. The sea is where you can go to learn to go with the flow, to be washed of your toxins, and to reconnect with your creative essence.

Going with the Flow

Water covers nearly three quarters of the surface of the earth and is necessary for the existence of life of all creatures on the planet. Water takes the shape of its container, be it the bed of an ocean, the bowl of a lake, or a simple drinking glass. It flows in the direction of gravity, and is pulled by the tides of the moon. These qualities are symbolic of going with the flow, moving with grace and ease, and being able to adapt to circumstances presented. As a human infant is made up of about eighty percent water (which diminishes over time to about fifty percent by age sixty or seventy), it is much more adaptable and resilient to circumstances. Its physiological and energetic make-up is much more fluid.

What Goes Around Comes Around - Cycles

The water cycle: evaporation, condensation, and precipitation, is symbolic of all things in life being cyclical in nature. The water cycle is a concrete example of the spiritual belief "what goes around comes around," that all things move in cycles, in processes, and eventually return to a beginning. The seasons that result from the evolution of the earth around the sun (spring, summer, autumn, and winter) are cyclical in nature as is the evolution process. The cycle of day to night that occurs as a result of the rotation of the earth on its axis is cyclical in nature. All things on the planet come and go and return from whence they came. The cyclical process of water reminds you to trust in the process of all things to come and go in flow.

Baptism and Spiritual Purification

Water rituals, such as baptism, are performed as a means of renewal and purification. The word baptism is derived from the Greek root word meaning "to wash." Just as water cleanses a wound or washes away a toxin physically, water is used energetically and spiritually to wash away demons and evil. What results is a state of cleanliness and purification in the eyes of Spirit, and a renewal to or reunion with the spiritual source. From a more practical standpoint, water can be used in your life as a means of washing away any energy that you deem no longer necessary or that has gone stagnant in your life.

Emotional Balance - Joy/Guilt

A healthy and balanced sacral chakra manifests in a healthy relationship with joy and guilt in your life.

The light emotion of the sacral chakra is joy. It governs all things in our lives that surround the concepts of pleasure, such as play, fun, creativity, adventure, and exploration. A balanced sacral chakra supports a healthy work/play balance, an ability and propensity for creativity and joy.

The shadow of the sacral chakra is guilt. When we are overwhelmed and feel we cannot live up to responsibility, guilt results. On some level, guilt is a healthy and necessary emotion because it keeps us in check and helps to make sure we are responsible and getting done what needs to get done. However, excessive guilt can quickly develop into a rigid and strict life without much room for play, pleasure, or joy, which is indication of an imbalance of the sacral chakra.

When your sacral chakra is balanced, you feel happy and joyful in all that you do, whether you are at work or at play. Guilt kicks in to remind you to be responsible and do what needs to get done even if it isn't all fun and games.

Characteristics of Imbalance

Excessive Sacral Chakra

An excessive sacral chakra means too much focus in life is put upon play, joy, pleasure, creativity, sexuality, adventure, and exploration. (How can this be a negative thing?) Symptoms may include:

> over-flexibility & hyperextension of joints
> drug addiction
> alcoholism
> pornography or sexual addiction
> excessive risk-taking
> excessive travel
> irresponsibility
> inability to focus or get things done
> inability to hold a job
> lack of muscle control

In today's modern society where 'sex sells' we are bombarded with images playing at the excessive sacral chakra constantly through advertising and marketing for whatever new pleasure is the next "must have."

Deficient Sacral Chakra

A deficient sacral chakra means not enough focus in life is given to pleasure, joy, play, adventure, creativity, vacations, enjoyment, and happiness. Symptoms may include:

workaholism
perfectionism
tight joints
feeling stuck
feeling overwhelmed
dryness or dehydration
inability to "go with the flow" (stubbornness)
lack of creativity
inability to laugh, smile, or have fun
sexual dysfunction or disinterest
anal-retentiveness
obsessive-compulsivity
problems with reproductive system organs
constipation

A great metaphor to describe someone with a deficient sacral chakra is to think of them as a tree or plant that hasn't received enough water and has become brittle and stiff.

Extreme Sacral Chakra

An extreme sacral chakra means that energy shifts from too much focus on work to complete irresponsibility. All work and no play makes for a very serious existence, but if you live in that for too long, eventually the pressure of an overburdened life builds up and requires a release, which in the case of an extreme sacral chakra results in extreme play. As an example, in an effort to maintain balance, someone with an extreme sacral chakra may work eighteen hour days for several weeks and then one day just decide not to show up for work and instead go on a five day party binge in Las Vegas. Symptoms may include:

- closeted sexually deviant behavior
- workaholism followed by irresponsible behaviors
- binge drinking or partying after stressful situations

The extreme sacral chakra is very difficult to balance. A great example of extreme sacral chakra imbalance is when a child becomes famous at a very young age and grows up working on movie and television sets or on music tours. They are constantly "on the job." Although the fame and fortune is fun, the demanding schedule, heavy workload, and burdens of responsibility take a toll on them. When they eventually reach adulthood age where they are legally of age to make decisions for themselves, they often revert to immaturity and irresponsibility, particularly in the form of addiction to drugs and alcohol and extreme partying with their millions of dollars.

Sacral Chakra Dominance

A dominant sacral chakra means that you have particular skill and talent in the areas of creativity, artistry, entertainment, play, adventure, exploration, and joy. These individuals have an innate ability to make others laugh and smile. People who have a dominant sacral chakra are exceptional at making others feel at happy, creative and adventurous.

Careers that are sacral chakra dominant include:

       entertainers
       musicians
       actors
       comedians
       artists
       writers
       inventors
       tour guides

Life Lesson - Go with the Flow

Aesop's Fable

The Oak and the Reeds

A mighty oak tree was uprooted by a gale and fell across a stream into some reeds. "How have you reeds, so frail, survived, when I, so strong, have been felled:" asked the oak tree. "You were stubborn and wouldn't bend," replied the reeds, "whereas we yield and allow the gale to pass harmlessly by."

Moral: go with the flow; better bend than to break

In this story, the strong solid oak tree falls while the pliable reeds survive the strong wind, the lesson being that survival is just as dependent upon flexibility and pliability as it is on strength and stability. As the reed did in this story, one must be able to 'go with the flow.' If you were to study the root system of reeds, you would see that it has a very dense root system, thus it is just as supported and solid as the oak tree, just not as solid and strong.

When the sacral chakra is imbalanced, the lessons that result are about going with the flow of life and being able to bend rather than break when certain challenges and gusts come your way. In many cases, going with the flow and bending to situations can provide new insights and visions that cannot be seen by the stubborn and solid. A balanced sacral chakra is both supported by its dense root system and pliable by its ability to find ease and grace no matter what comes your way.

Balancing Practices & Prescriptions

Diet & Nutrition

A **deficient sacral chakra** is dehydrated, thus drinking more water will help hydrate the sacral chakra. Foods that are exceptionally juicy, such as citrus fruits, tomatoes, cucumbers, zucchini, and more will increase the fluidity in your system. Any food that leaves a significant puddle on your cutting board will help nourish the deficient sacral chakra. Adding healthy fats and oils in moderation, such as avocados and olive oil will provide lubrication to your joints. Supplementing with omega 3 fatty acids will also support a deficient sacral chakra. Furthermore, since a deficient sacral chakra results in workaholism and perfectionism, which often develop in an overall sense of uptightness, small doses of alcohol can help loosen up the rigidity. 1-2 glasses of wine each week can make a huge difference for sacral chakra deficiency.

Since an **excessive sacral chakra** often manifests into addiction, cutting out addictive substances is necessary. Quite often someone with an excessive sacral chakra is lacking in basic nutrition. Basic nutrition is the result of a consistent discipline, which is an antidote for the excessive sacral chakra. Replacing junk foods with a healthy balance of fruits, vegetables, proteins, and grains can provide the discipline and consistency necessary to treat sacral excess.

The **extreme sacral chakra** swings from flood to drought, so consistency is key. Quite often, an extreme sacral chakra goes from a strict rigid diet to a complete disregard for health and nutrition, or from complete abstinence from something like alcohol or sugar to over-indulgence. The dietary key to balance is to never deny yourself of anything, but to allow yourself everything, including junk foods and alcoholic beverages in small moderate doses. For example, for every glass of wine you have, drink 2-3 times as much plain water.

Body Mechanics - Joints

From the smallest joint of your baby toe to the intricate joints in your spine to the large ball and socket joint of your hips, your joints provide your physical body with flexibility, giving you the ability to move and flow in various degrees and directions. Hyperextension of the joints results in hyper-flexibility, excessive sacral chakra. Rigidity of the joints results in inflexibility, deficient sacral chakra. Learning proper body mechanics of your joints, with both stability and flexibility, promotes the balance of your sacral chakra. Stability and flexibility are apparent opposites, but this dual action, when engaged simultaneously within the human body, help access a sensation deep inside the tissues that support centering and u balance.

Try this exercise: reach your arms as far forward as you can, pushing through your palms as if you are reaching for a wall to support you. This tests the full range of motion of your shoulder joints and how your arms interact with your shoulder girdle and chest. As you do this test, pay attention to where you feel the stretch in your back, chest and arms.. What you may notice is that the muscles that are stretched are closer to the skin on your back and your outside arms. What you have done is lengthened these muscles to their fullest extent. If you were to try to hold a weight in your hands at this full extension, chances are, these same muscles, closer to the skin, will fatigue relatively quickly. In order to achieve full range of motion or flexibility, some strength and stability is compromised and sacrificed.

Try this same exercise again, but this time, from a place of stability. Lift your arms up, pushing away from you. Instead of reaching or pushing your palms forward, plug your arm bones back into socket. You may notice similar muscles in your back and arms engage, but this time they feel strong instead of long. What you have done is shortened the length of the muscle. If you were to try to hold a weight in your hands, the stability of your muscles would allow you to last longer, with less fatigue. In this case, you have sacrificed flexibility for stability and strength.

Try one more time, but this time, first plug your arms into your shoulder sockets, while keeping that stability engaged, push the palms of your hands forward. Take note of what you feel in your muscles. Chances are, you will still feel the muscles across your back and the outside of your arms. However, this time you may also feel muscles deeper inside your body, closer to your heart and spine, engage and stretch. You may even feel muscles engage down into your core. What you have done by the dual action of stability and flexibility is to bring the work of the exercise deeper inside the tissues of your body and redistribute the effort of the action across more muscles of your body.

Another way to think of this exercise is to apply it to lifting a heavy box from the floor. If you bend over at your waist to lift the box, you are going into full flexibility of the muscles around your low back and backs of your legs, which lessens your strength and stability and puts you at deeper risk for injuries such as pulled muscles or compressed discs. However, if you squat down, you are stabilizing the joints of your low back and hips first and then allowing the strength of the deeper muscles of your legs and bum to support the weight. Not only is the box easier to lift, you are less likely to injure yourself.

Energetically, this physical action of stabilizing your joints before stretching them serves as a link from chakra to chakra, allowing the energy to flow like water between and amongst several chakras at once, rather than isolating the action. Working the body as a whole rather than separate individual units is called functional unity.

Exercise

Swimming, kayaking, canoeing, paddle boarding, surfing, and other water sports can help balance the sacral chakra because they all teach you to both respect the immense power of water and to remember that your own body is made up of more than half water. Learning to work with the power and flow of water, yet control it just enough to not be overwhelmed or overtaken by it is exceptionally healing for the sacral chakra.

While water sports are excellent forms of exercise for the sacral chakra, they are sometimes very impractical. However, since the human body is over 50% water, working the body in ways that move the fluids through your system is also healing. Dancing is one easy way to do this. Another way is through flowing yoga, which is a style of yoga that means to move fluidly from one position to another, and in many ways, it looks like dancing.

Breathing Practice - Cooling Breath

A simple way to bring more fluidity into your system is to breathe it in over your tongue. When you inhale through your tongue as a straw, tiny droplets of water off your tongue evaporate into the air that passes into your lungs, serving as a natural vaporizer. Breathe out through your nose, so as not to allow liquid to escape off your tongue. Then, curl your tongue and inhale through the straw of your tongue. When you do this, notice the temperature change of the air as it passes over your tongue, it is cooler, and it is more humid. This cool humidity serves to soothe and calm your system, as water does naturally.

Elemental Practices - Water

Children love to engage with water as a pleasurable activity. From swimming to water slides, water pistols to running through the sprinkle, tossing water balloons to jumping in puddles, a good splash always brings a giggle and a smile to a child. This is because water is the ultimate healer. It cleanses and washes away the debris. It dilutes the intense and cools the heat. People engage in simple water rituals to provide energetic healing of the sacral chakra on a daily basis.

Cleansing

Water is the first line of defense against all toxins, physical and energetic. The simple practice of washing your hands regularly to wash away bacteria is a great defense against viruses and infections, both physical and energetic. When you encounter people or situations that challenge your sacral chakra energy of joy and pleasure and send you into toxicity or anger or frustration, a good dose of water can be excellent medicine. If you feel overworked, overwhelmed, or overburdened, a good long shower or hot bath always soothes the muscles and emotions and washes away the tensions and frustrations. Next time you encounter a toxic situation or someone who zaps you of your joy and pleasure, try washing it off, literally, by washing your hands and face. Chances are, you'll feel better.

Diluting

When we add water to things, it dilutes the potency or intensity of the liquid. Water will do the same thing for energies and situations. If things feel rather intense, or too dense, or a little too potent, try drinking water, or adding a water fountain to the space, or turning on the faucet, or taking a shower. A good walk by a river or in the rain without an umbrella will quickly dilute anything that is too intense and offer you a cooler and cleaner perspective on the situation or circumstance.

Cooling

When tensions rise, and particularly when situations get heated, the cooling element of water can quickly smooth and calm any situation. If you encounter a particularly angry person or heated situation, try drinking water or going to the bathroom to wash your hands and face. The water will cool off any over-heated tensions.

Mindful Concentration Techniques

The following prescriptions are more spiritually based practices that are balancing and healing for the sacral chakra.

- Meditating on the color ORANGE
- Offering gratitude to WATER
- Chanting the sacral chakra seed sound VAM
- Visualizing your own FLUIDITY

Journaling Topics

1. Where do you feel 'stuck' in your life? In what areas of your life are you unwilling or unable to 'go with the flow'?

2. What are you holding onto in life that needs to be released? What issues need to become 'water under the bridge' so you can move on with your life?

3. What things in your life have served their purpose but have stuck around to become toxic? Examples are toxic relationships, toxic situations, addictions, and unhealthy behaviors.

4. Are you a workaholic? When do you tend to get overwhelmed with burden and responsibility? Are you a perfectionist? Do you take your jobs and responsibilities so seriously that you don't know how to relax?

5. When was the last time you had a good laugh? What makes you feel joy and pleasure? What can you do to bring more ease, grace, joy and flow into your daily routine?

6. Do you tend towards partying? Do you drink or use sex or drugs to "get away from it all" or to escape your reality? Why or how do you depend on things outside yourself to escape or bring you pleasure and joy?

CHAPTER 6

The Core Chakra

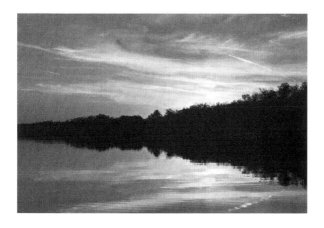

Sanskrit - Manipura

Mani = Precious Gem
Pura = Fulfilling

Definition

The manipura, located in the center of the abdomen is the home to your gut instinct. It is the center of your sense of purpose and power. Think of it as the precious gem of your being, held by the cushion of the soft tissues of your abdomen.

Governing Realm - Personal Power

Career
Personal Power
Life Purpose
Identity
Individuality
Passion & Drive
Motivation

The power of the core chakra is Personal Power, governing drive, passion, motivation, strength, confidence, self-esteem, individuality, uniqueness, identity, life purpose, and career. A balanced core chakra supports a healthy sense of self. You know who you are, and you have a healthy sense of self worth.

Body Location - Torso & Abdomen

The body part connected to the core chakra is the torso, including your digestive organs and your abdominal muscles. Typically, we think of the core muscles as the abdominal muscles, the superficial muscles surrounding your belly, those muscles closest to the skin. While physical fitness trainers often teach about engaging the core muscles, and images of six-pack abs are considered highly attractive in modern culture, the muscles that support the core chakra are deeper inside the body. To really feel your core chakra, you must connect with the muscles deeper in your abdomen. These muscles are the psoas and the diaphragm, which intertwine with each other. The psoas muscles connect your lower body with your upper body to create the effect that your body moves as one unit. In essence, the psoas and diaphragm are the stitching that hold your body together at its center.

The psoas muscles are a group of muscles that connect the inside of your thigh bones through your pelvis to the inside of both hip bones and then continue on up to your lumbar vertebrae and the vertebrae that connect to your lower ribs. These are the only muscles that weave through the pelvis and connect the upper body to the lower body.

Think of the psoas muscles as a straw, or tubular channel that transmit energy between the upper and lower body. As you learned in chapter three, the root chakra draws energy from Mother Earth through the conscious placement of your feet and the activation of your inner thigh muscles (adductors). The psoas muscles connect directly to the inner thighs and continue the process of drawing nourishment from Mother Earth into the rest of the body, specifically by connecting to the ribs and thus the lungs and heart where all energies are dispersed through the body.

Going in the other direction, the psoas muscles can transmit energy from the heart and lungs of the upper body through the pelvis to the lower body. When you breathe deep into your back ribs, your psoas muscles get tugged like rubber-bands. Because they are connected to the inner thigh, they then tug on the femur bone, serving as a channel to bring energy from your lungs into your legs and feet.

Because the psoas muscles are buried deep inside the center of your body, it is also easy to compress and constrict them, thus restricting the flow of energy. Proper alignment of your torso, from the base of your hips to the top of your ribs allows for optimal channeling of energy. When these muscles are bent, compressed, or folded, energy flow lessens, which then requires you to use other muscles to perform tasks. Your psoas muscles are strong and free, and because they are buried so deep inside your system, connecting you to the core of your being, they support the functioning of your body and your life from your center.

Your diaphragm is a large muscle that lines the lower lip of your rib cage, all the way around from front to back. It serves as a partition between the thoracic cavity, containing the heart and lungs, and the abdominal cavity, containing the digestive organs. The diaphragm is as vital as the lungs to the breathing function. When lifted it looks like the top of an inflated balloon, which compresses the lungs and forces air out. When lowered it looks like a floor to the ribcage, which opens space for the lungs to expand and take in air.

The diaphragm is also used to control the movement of fluids. It is one of the primary muscles used to expel vomit, feces, and urine from the body. Thus, the diaphragm physiologically helps us to get rid of what we no longer need. Furthermore, if you think of the acidic juices of your stomach as fire, the diaphragm also serves to control the fire of your body by keeping pressure and a wall between the digestive organs and the breathing organs of your body.

The psoas muscles and the diaphragm muscle weave together right at the center of your physical body, serving as a basket of strength and flexibility. The core chakra, your precious gem, is held by the interweaving of the psoas and diaphragm muscles. Its energy is then transmitted through the rest of the body through this pairing of significant muscle groups.

Development Stage - Pre-School

The core chakra develops during the time of pre-school and kindergarten, roughly between the ages of two and five years of age. The balance of your core chakra is somewhat connected to what was happening in your life during your pre-school years, particularly in your ability to develop your identity, assert your own personal power, and be valued for your individuality. To gain a better understanding of the development of your core chakra, take some time to contemplate the following during the time of your preschool years:

1. Opportunities you were given to make your own decisions and choices
2. Particular likes and dislikes you started asserting at a young age and how those were received by people close to you
3. Whether you parents encouraged you to do things yourself or did things for you when you were young. What things were you allowed to do for yourself and what things were you not allowed to do?

4. Your family's tendencies towards confidence, strength, power, will, drive, motivation, passion, enthusiasm, etc.
5. Any friendships you may have had that played out the roles of victim or bully.
6. Your self-esteem as a child and how your family supported your sense of identity.

Independence

Children at the age of 3 to 5 usually start saying to their parents that they can "do it themselves" and want to start taking care of their own needs in many ways. This is the age when children start to learn to dress themselves, to brush their own teeth, eventually tie their own shoes, and maybe even ride a bike. As coordination is developing in both gross and fine motor skills, children at this age are discovering a new sense of independence. Play at this age often involves mimicking adult behavior, such as playing house or copying adult-like behavior with action figures, dolls, or barbies.

If you were encouraged to take initiative and your sense of independence was fostered at this age, this helped develop your core chakra and your sense of confidence and self-sufficiency. Did the adults in your life encourage you to make your own choices and decisions? Did they value your opinions, even though you were young? Or did they make most of your decisions for you? Did they teach you how to do things and patiently wait while you figured out how to accomplish tasks, or did they often get impatient and just do things for you instead? If you were coddled or overly pampered or enabled as a child, particularly during your pre-school years, your core chakra development may have been stunted.

Identity

Pre-school is when children start to go through phases, particularly in asserting their individual likes and dislikes. For example, their eating often gets much more finicky as they assert that they love macaroni and cheese but won't even touch a meatball. While phases come and go, they are healthy expressions of exploring their own identities and desires. Parents of pre-school age children start to recognize their child's individual personality quirks and character traits.

These phases and expressions of personality and character are healthy indications of core chakra development. Each phase is like trying on a piece of energetic clothing to see what fits and feels good and what doesn't. Some phases last longer than others. Some phases stick, like the clothing you choose to buy and take home. Other phases become a staple in your life, like that favorite sweater that you have worn every winter since you were fifteen.

Personal Power

If you ever take some time to watch pre-school age children play, there is often a power-struggle at play. As pre-school children are starting to recognize their identity in relationships with others, they are testing the boundaries of their personal power through play. Some children become bossy while others become followers. Sometimes these roles change significantly based on different scenarios. For example, a follower on the playground with peers may become a bully with her younger siblings at home. Oftentimes these behaviors manifest in scolding from adults and children learn the emotions of guilt and shame as a means of understanding where the line is between personal power and bullying.

Essentially, at this age the core chakra is pulsating between excessive and deficient in an effort to find what fits just right for itself. When children behave as bossy bullies and then are reprimanded and told they are "bad kids" because of their behavior, the shame kicks in and they swing from the excessive bully to the deficient "I'm not good" energy of the core chakra. A healthy core chakra develops when the child learns the balance between standing in their own identity without suppressing the power and identity of others.

Self-Esteem

As pre-school children are exploring their own identities, this is also when their self-esteem develops. An exceptionally high self-esteem is a sense of confidence and self-worth, while a low self-esteem is a feeling of not being good enough. Too much self-esteem can be too prideful, while not enough can manifest into victimization and inferiority.

If children in pre-school are taught and validated for their inherent goodness and their individuality a healthy balance of the core chakra results. However, western culture puts so much value on competition and superiority that valuing each individual for their own gifts and talents is difficult to do without comparison and ranking. As early as pre-school age popular educational television shows like *Sesame Street* teach and encourage children to categorize things as good or bad, best or worst. The world is dualistic, and it is human nature to want to compare things to each other. But when comparison pertains to the inherent value of a person, self-esteem is challenged and the core chakra development is impacted.

A healthy self-esteem, and thus a healthy and balanced core chakra, is when you know and value the inherent goodness within yourself regardless of what other people say about you and how they treat you. In addition, a healthy and balanced self-esteem recognizes your humanity and is able to handle emotions of shame and guilt as signals that you are not behaving in a manner that reflects and values the inherent goodness in yourself.

Ecological Element - Fire

The element for the core chakra is FIRE, symbolic of passion, drive, motivation, power, and endurance. Fire is hot, igniting, inciting, instigating, and consuming.

Energy

Fire is necessary for the fundamental sustenance of life, particularly for its energy producing qualities. From small indigenous tribal villages to the largest of industrial societies, fire provides necessary energy for survival. We burn coal, oil, gas, and wood to produce heat for our homes just as campfires and village fires provide heat in the elements of nature. Food is cooked over fire, eaten, and then digested. The digestive process involves the burning or oxidization (fire) of the food to produce energy for our muscles, organs, and tissues.

Alchemical Transformation

When fire burns something, that something is chemically transformed from its current state into energy, smoke and ash. The smoke rises up into the air and gets absorbed by the atmosphere while the ash is absorbed by the earth and serves an important role as fertilizer to new growth. When forest fires consume the natural growth of the land, what remains is ash, which then nourishes the soil for fresh new growth, as is part of the cycle of life. Fire is often what is used to consume and kill that which no longer serves and to change its form into something that serves.

A common spiritual practice is a burning bowl ceremony where you write down all the things in your life that you are ready to have changed and transformed, those things that no longer serve you in their current state, and to burn them. Many people find themselves having fires to symbolically burn away the past and start new. Within your own body, at the center of your core chakra, you body has an internal fire (digestive juices and enzymes) that burns up the food you eat as fuel and transform it into cells that nourish your body and provide you with energy to serve the functions you need to engage in the world.

Energetically, from the chakra perspective, fire is the element within your core chakra that burns up all that is not true to your identity in order to provide fuel and energy for the manifestation of your independence and personal power.

Smoke

Smoke is used in many traditions as a spiritual cleansing agent. Whether you are smudging yourself to clean your aura or using burning sage or lemongrass or incense to cleanse a space, or burning a scented candle to change the aroma (and energy) of a room, the quality of smoke is to absorb the dense energy that is no longer needed and take it away into the atmosphere.

Unconsciously, when someone takes a smoke-break they are energetically inhaling a small kick of energy, both in the stimulant characteristics of the nicotine as well as the energetic quality of fire. Many people who are overworked, over-stimulated, and living in high-stress situations that require high-energy are drawn to smoking as a means of getting energy.

Candlelight Vigils

Candlelight vigils are a means of connecting with loved ones who have died. Whether you are lighting a candle for your ancestors at an altar at church or holding vigil at the site of a tragedy, the fire is symbolic of transformation of the loved one from the physical to the spiritual realm, as in alchemical process described above. The vigil is a way of recognizing and honoring the power, identity and individuality (core chakra) of the individual who has transformed from the physical to the spirit.

Emotional Balance - Power & Shame

A healthy and balanced core chakra manifests in a healthy relationship with power and shame in your life.

The light emotion of the core chakra is power. It governs all things in our lives that surround the concepts of power, strength, identity, purpose, drive, motivation, and confidence. A balanced core chakra supports a healthy self-esteem and confidence in your own strength, gifts, talents, and abilities.

The shadow emotion of the core chakra is shame. When we behave in ways that are not in alignment with our authentic sense of self, with who we really are and how we want to present ourselves to the world, shame manifests. In addition, if we act in a way that is not respectful to others and their gifts, talents and authenticity, we feel shame. On some level, shame is a healthy and necessary emotion because it keeps us in check and helps to make sure we are acting in accordance to our true nature and respectful of others in the same way. Excessive shame can quickly develop into weakness while a lack of shame can develop into narcissism.

When your sacral chakra is balanced, you feel happy and joyful in all that you do, whether you're at work or at play. Guilt kicks in to remind you to be responsible and do what needs to get done even if it isn't all fun and games.

Characteristics of Imbalance

Excessive Core Chakra

An excessive core chakra means congested energy in the areas of power, strength, identity, and motivation. Symptoms may include:

> bullying
> stubbornness
> lack of compassion
> an inability to relate to others
> bossiness
> inflexibility
> ulcers
> acid reflux
> over-protectiveness

Deficient Core Chakra

A deficient core chakra is lacking energy in the core chakra in the areas of independence, individuality, personal power, and motivation. Symptoms may include:

> victimization

weakness - both physical and emotional
Wimpy
low self-esteem
poor digestive functioning
lack of motivation, apathy
sluggishness or laziness
exhaustion or sense of complete depletion
dependence upon others
anorexia or under-eating

Extreme Core Chakra

An extreme sacral chakra means that energy shifts from victim to bully, energetic to fatigue, depending upon the situation and circumstance at hand.

all or nothing attitude
adrenal exhaustion
bullying

Core Chakra Dominance

A dominant core chakra means that you have particular skill and talent in the areas of empowerment, individuality, uniqueness, strength, confidence, motivation, drive, and passion. These individuals have an innate ability to empower others. Careers that are sacral chakra dominant include:

lawyers
corporate executives
marketing specialists
fitness trainers and body builders
athletes

Life Lessons - Hold Your Power

Aesop's Fable

The Horse, Hunter, and Stag

A quarrel had arisen between the Horse and the Stag, so the Horse came to a Hunter to ask his help to take revenge on the Stag. The Hunter agreed, but said: "If you desire to conquer the Stag, you must permit me to place this piece of iron between your jaws, so that I may guide you with these reins, and allow this saddle to be placed upon your back so that I may keep steady upon you as we follow after the enemy." The Horse agreed to the conditions, and the Hunter soon saddled and bridled him. Then with the aid of the Hunter the Horse soon overcame the Stag, and said to the Hunter: "Now, get off, and remove those things from my mouth and back."

"Not so fast, friend," said the Hunter. "I have now got you under bit and spur, and prefer to keep you as you are at present."

If you allow men to use you for your own purposes, they will use you for theirs.

In this story, the quarrel between the Horse and the Stag are symbolic of two core chakras in competition with each other. Rather than valuing each other for their innate gifts and unique differences, they argue. In an effort to assert power over the Stag, the Horse enlists the help of the Hunter, who convinces the Horse to relinquish power. The story is an example of how competition causes imbalances in power and pits energies against each other rather than working in cooperation. Essentially, the Horse gave away his own power in an effort to assert power over the Stag. In the end, none of the individuals in the story is really standing in his power, but instead are participating in a tug of war of power against each other.

The lesson here lies in holding your own power while also honoring the power of others. Each person you meet has gifts and talents, as do you. When you honor those gifts and talents, especially if you do not share them in yourself, you are honoring the value of individuality that each being has something unique and honorable to contribute to the good of the whole.

Balancing Practices & Prescriptions

Diet & Nutrition

A **deficient core chakra** is like a fire that is dying out, a wood-burning stove that needs fuel. In extreme cases, when a fire is dying an accelerant is necessary to get the wood to light again. Dietarily, a kick of spicy food (ginger, jalapeños, chili powder, crushed red pepper, chiles, etc.) can be just the kick you need to light your fire. Nibbling quarter size slice of fresh ginger after each meal freshens your breath, clears you palate, aids in digestion, and gives your energetic fuel a little kick. Remember, ecologically the sun is very far away and a little bit of fire goes a very long way. Take spicy foods in moderation!

An **excessive core chakra** is one with too much heat, too much fire. When fires get too hot, they consume and dry up everything around them. Again water is key. Drink more water, just plain water. Coffee is not water. Tea is not water, even watered down juice is not water. Drink water, 8-10 glasses of plain water per day. Secondly, stop adding fuel to the fire by eliminating or reducing spicy and heating foods from your diet. Also, avoid eating dehydrating foods (coffee, tea, alcohol, dried foods) that will suck the fluid out of your system. Finally, if you tend toward an exceptionally hot temper and over-consuming fire, adding dairy such as milk, cream, and yogurt, can quickly soothe the excess heat and provide the energy of compassion to your system.

The **extreme core chakra** swings from hot to cold. Balance is lacking. Try consuming food and water that are room temperature. Avoid extreme diets such as Indian and Mexican. The Indians offer extremely spicy foods and then balance them with extreme cooling foods like cucumber and yogurt sauce, while Mexican food balances the spice with lots of cooling sour cream and cheese.

Body Mechanics - Core Embrace

Looking at the human torso without the skin, the muscles of the torso (psoas, diaphragm, abdominals, obliques) form a sort of ace-bandage criss-crossing and wrapping around the entire mid-section of the body. Furthermore, this part of the body has only the vertebrae at the back body as bones to hold the structure of the body. Thus, the engagement of these muscles is necessary to the support and protection of the vital organs of the digestive and reproductive systems.

From an energetic perspective, the core embrace is like a gentle hug of your core chakra, your precious gem. If your core chakra holds your personal power and your identity, your sense of self, the core embrace is a means of hugging that sense of self, of embracing your individuality and holding your personal power.

Core embrace is not be confused with a stiff and rigorous engagement of your belly muscles. While you do want these muscles engaged, you also want enough space, fluidity and ease in your core to move freely from one position to another. Core embrace is a means of gently activating all of your core muscles appropriately to support your core. It is common to over-engage the abdominal muscles (those used to perform sit-ups) and let the others slack, particularly the interior muscles of the psoas and diaphragm. In fact, core embrace feels like a slight lifting in and up from deep inside your torso.

1. Stand up against a wall as if you are being measured for height. In fact, you may even ask someone to measure your height as a pre-test. Then, use your hand or fist to measure the space between your low back and the wall. Take note of how much space is there.

2. Place your feet and activate your adductor muscles as described in the root chakra chapter. The top of your adductor muscles connect with the bottom of your psoas muscles on your upper thigh bone. So, when you activate your adductor muscles, they give your psoas muscles a little message to engage as well. You may notice that when you squeeze a yoga block between your thighs, you feel a slight engagement in your lower belly. This is your third chakra, core embrace, beginning to activate.

3. Place your thumbs on your lower ribs and your middle fingers on the tip of your hip bones and gently pull them slightly closer to each other, just a little 'titch' that drops your pelvis and lifts your inner core. You may feel that inner belly muscle get a little stronger and lift slightly.

4. Measure the space behind your back once again. Chances are, it is slightly less. If you have your friend re-measure your height, you may have grown a few centimeters, or even more! With core embrace, people often report a feeling of being more confident, stronger, taller, and lighter.

Let's take this experiment into motion. Take a little stroll around the room, just walking as you normally would. Pay special attention to what you are looking at and how your body feels, including the weight of your arms and legs and the sensations in your torso. Then, stop and activate the core embrace as described in the previous paragraph. Keep that core embrace and take the same walk around the room. Notice your walking posture and become aware of how you feel. Do you notice any difference or change?

Most people report that they find that with the core embrace, they are looking straight ahead rather than down at their feet, they feel like they are walking taller, and their limbs feel lighter and easier to move. Some people even report that the core embrace gives them the feeling of floating.

When you have core embrace properly engaged, you may feel like a floating and upward lifting from your center. When this upward lifting occurs, you upper body is free and light. This means that your breath is free, your arms are lighter, and your head and shoulders are relaxed.

Exercise

Strength training is an excellent form of exercise that supports the core chakra. Weight lifting, which often creates a slight burning sensation in the muscles, produces a heat building effect from the inside out. Plyometrics and isometric stretches also produce heat building energy to support the core chakra. Any core strengthening exercises such as Pilates, power yoga or sit-ups help as well. Try any form of exercise that is heat-building and causes a subtle burning sensation in the muscles and produces sweat, such as cardiovascular exercises, aerobic fitness, weight training, interval training, and more.

Be careful not to overdo any heat-building exercise as it is easy to burn-out and cause fatigue or to injure muscles by overuse or over-exertion. A little bit of heat goes a long way, which is why the sun, our primary source of heat, is very far away.

Breathing Practice - Breath of Fire

When you fan a flame, the fire burns brighter and stronger, so when you add air to the internal heater of your body, you will stoke the energetic fire of your system. Your digestive system is where your fuel is processed, and the home to firey enzymes and acids to burn that fuel. Thus, the home of your internal heater is in your abdomen, so belly breathing is much like using a bellows on the fire of a wood-burning stove.

Take a deep breath in through your nose, and then, in short even bursts, pull the muscles of your abdomen in towards your spine. Each belly thrust creates a vacuum effect and forces air out through your mouth. Several quick breaths (20-30) at a time will both exercise the muscles of your abdomen and massage the energetic home of your core chakra. With this kind of breath, focus only on the exhale as the vacuum effect with automatically create an inhale. After a few rounds, you may even find yourself sweating.

Elemental Practices - Fire

Ecologically, the sun is the ultimate source of energy. When the sun is up and bright, we are active and alert, busy and motivated. Whereas, on dreary days or during the darkness of night, we tend more towards lethargy and restfulness. We use the energy fire in many ways, to cook our food, to warm our bodies and environments, and in spiritual practices to connect with spirit.

Warming

As a general rule, most liquids flow more freely when they are warm. Thus, because your body is made up mostly of fluid, when it is warm, it is much easier to move and be active. In any exercise class, a warm-up session is necessary to properly and safely prepare the muscles for the intense work of the fitness routine. The heat of fire, be it produced by the sun, by burning something, or by friction and movement, gets the juices flowing and supports ease in activity and movement. When you need to get going, motivation to move, a little ignition of fire through a good warm-up will support you.

Igniting

When we want to start something new, like starting a car, we need to turn on the "ignition" which simply means lighting the fire. Other words or phrases of getting something going include spark, light a fire underneath, or turn on the heat. Any form of fuel, be it coal or natural gas or food in our stomachs, is burned to produce energy. If you need a kick of motivation to get something going, lighting a candle, turning up the heat, to producing friction through movement in your body will give you that motivation. Ironically, even smoking cigarettes can be a motivational kick. Often smokers find energy from a cigarette because they are not only bringing the quality of fire into their bodies, they are breathing deep. This is not to advocate smoking because the negative effects of nicotine and tar build-up on the lungs are not worth the energetic benefits. However, everything has its pros and cons.

Spiritual Rituals

At many churches, candles are lit as a means of connecting with Spirit or honoring our deceased loved ones. Fire has long been used in spiritual traditions as a means of connecting with Spirit or cleansing a spiritual space. Burning incense, sage, or lemongrass can transform the energy of a space just as it transforms the element being burned into smoke and ash. A lit candle can serve as a gateway between the physical world and the spiritual world where it is commonly believed is the home of our deceased loved ones.

Mindful Concentration Techniques

The following prescriptions are more spiritually based practices that are balancing and healing for the core chakra.

1. Meditating on the color YELLOW
2. Offering gratitude to FIRE
3. Sacred FIRES in which you burn away what you no longer need and make space for something new.
4. Chanting the sacral chakra seed sound RAM
5. Visualizing your own FIRE at the center of your belly
6. Candlelight VIGILS

Journaling Topics

1. Where do you feel 'stuck' in your life? In what areas of your life are you unable to get going and need a kick of motivation or inspiration or ignition?
2. What are you holding onto in life that needs to be released? What issues do you need to burn away to make space for something new?
3. What things in your life have served their purpose but have stuck around to become toxic and now need to be burned out? This includes but not be limited to toxic relationships, toxic situations, addictions, unhealthy behaviors, and more.
4. In what areas of your life have you overdone things and experienced a result of burn-out? Where do you have too much passion and drive and motivation that it eventually fizzles?
5. Do you tend to get great ideas and run with them for a short time, but eventually lose steam or burn-out? How do tend to light the fire too hot and then not have enough fuel for the endurance of what you want to do?
6. Do you tend to get lazy or lethargic and need a kick of motivation or drive?
7. When have you been bullied or victimized in your life? Have you ever been the bully? If yes, what drove you to that behavior? What could you do to balance your sense of personal power without burning out those people around you?

CHAPTER 7

The Heart Chakra

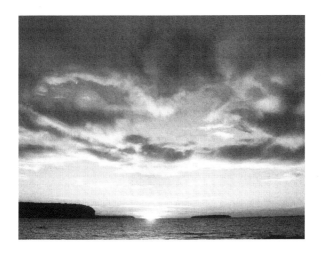

Sanskrit - Anahata

Ana = Not
Hata = Struck

Definition

The Anahata is the Heart Chakra. We think of the heart as the part of our being that gets broken when relationships come to an end. However, deep inside the heart is a beautiful space, where the two sides have one center, that space that is unable to be broken, the piece of ourselves that knows true love as unconditional.

Governing Realm - Love

Relationships
Romance
Giving & Receiving
Friendships
Love
Compassion
Self-Love

The power of the heart chakra is Love, governing love, relationships, friendships, romance, the balance between giving and receiving, compassion, and self-love. A balanced heart chakra supports healthy relationships with a good balance of give and take, share and receive.

Body Location - Chest & Arms

The body parts connected to the Heart Chakra are the chest and arms, including the shoulders, ribs, lungs, heart, arms and hands. The arms are what we use to interact with life, to do things. As the heart chakra is about love, particularly the giving and receiving of love, think of the arms as the physical expression of love. We use our arms to grasp and embrace as well as to give away and share. To become conscious and aware of how you hold your shoulders and arms is to become consciously aware of your ability to take in and experience life, and to let go of what you no longer need.

In today's world, it is common to spend much of the day slouched in front of computer screens, your upper back and shoulders taking the toll for the constant hunching over a keyboard. One of the most common places to hold stress and feel tight and restricted is through the upper back and shoulders. We think of our shoulders as burdening the "weight of the world" because they hold all the things that we take in and have difficulty eventually letting go. People carry an immense amount of stress in their shoulders, stress being worries and burdens and responsibilities. Our ability to take in what is ours, do what we need, and let go of that which is not ours and delegate what we need not do is tied up in the flexibility, strength, and tightness of our shoulders. If you take a deep breath, it is the exhalation that generally produces a wave of calm and peace throughout your system because it allows you to let go, to release the stresses and burdens that are no longer serving you.

On an energetic level, interacting with computer screens rather than real life greatly diminishes your ability to relate to others because the 'hugging muscles' of your arms and shoulders are so tight. When you slouch, your chest caves in, over-protecting the heart inside the ribcage. Over time, your neck can collapse, creating an action that is very much like a turtle pulling its head into its shell, which is symbolic of wanting to shut out others.

While your neck and lower back have natural curvature and flexibility in your spine, your middle back (thoracic spine) does not, partly because this part of your spine is connected to all your ribs limiting your flexibility in its effort to protect. Add to this anatomical fact the practicality of engaging in the world in front of you and the tendencies to hunch and slouch, and the thoracic spine becomes even more limited in its ability, particularly to bend backwards, to open your chest. As a result, your chest caves in more, causing a restriction in breath. Since breath is how you take in life and engage in the world around you, keeping this part of your body flexible so that you can breathe fully is vital to the fullest experience of life.

Backbends are a great way to increase the flexibility of your thoracic spine. However, it is easy to avoid the stretch of the upper middle back in favor of the more flexible neck and lower back, thus it is common to dump backbends into the lumbar spine or over-exert them from the neck. Your middle back, containing and protecting your heart is the backbone to sacred territory in your system, that part of you that is the most genuine, the most pure, your heart. In order to put your heart out there in the world, you must feel safe. If you don't feel safe, you are likely to protect your heart more and compromise the integrity of your body elsewhere, such as your neck or low back. Backbends need to be performed from leg strength because the legs are the place of the body where safety and security are protected.

Development Stage - Grade School

The heart chakra develops during the time of grade school, roughly between the ages of six to eleven years old. The balance of your heart chakra is somewhat connected to what was happening in your life during your grade school years, particularly in your ability to develop and maintain friendships, to establish healthy relationships on all levels, to facilitate a balance in your life between giving to others and receiving from others, and an ability to recover from loss and grief. To gain a better understanding of the development of your heart chakra, take some time to reflect and research the following during the time of your grade school years:

1. Friendships and relationships with your peers.
2. Relationships with adults and understanding and respect for authority without feelings of inferiority or victimization
3. Your ability to give and receive equally, sharing with others and allowing others to share with you
4. Your family's tendencies towards affection, love, connection, and relationships
5. Any traumas or tragedies in your life that resulted in the loss of a loved one, such as moving to a new home, death of a friend or family member, loss of a pet or other significant loss
6. Puppy love romances

Relationships

Remember the days of grade school, when you gave Valentine's cards to every single kid in class, even the ones you didn't particularly like? While peer groups start to form at this age, children still hold love and respect for everyone in their environments. They look up to all adults, and often idolize older siblings, recognizing the inherent good in all beings. In addition, this is the time when children start to collaborate in both play and education. From peer reading groups or collaborative math clubs to girl scouts and boy scouts and youth sports, children are developing their ability to work together and cooperate.

If you were encouraged to take part in cooperative activities in grade school such as scouting, youth sports, martial arts, and after school clubs, chances are that this helped your heart chakra develop and teach you how to relate to others in a variety of settings. Did the adults in your life encourage you to participate in activities that exposed you to a variety of people? Did they value diversity and encourage you to accept others unconditionally? Or, did they model judgmental behaviors? Were you exposed to discrimination and prejudice?

Love & Loss

Grade school is often the developmental period when children are old enough to experience and understand the effects of loss. Despite the measures adults take to shelter and protect children from the pains of loss and grief, inevitably, some trauma or tragedy occurs during grade school that exposes children to sorrow. Whether the loss is the death of a friend or family member, to passing of a beloved pet, the moving away of a good friend, children in grade school are mature enough to comprehend loss and experience grief, and it is part of the human experience.

When grief and loss came into your life during grade school, how the adults in your life supported you in processing the grief would have a direct impact on the development of the heart chakra. Were you overly protected and sheltered against exposure to loss? What significant loss or grief did you experience as a grade school aged child? Did the adults in your life listen to your concerns and allow you to express your sadness during times of loss, or did they encourage you to quickly get over it and move on?

Giving & Receiving

Grade school is when children learn the value of giving and receiving. Whether it be through birthday parties, valentines or holidays, children are encouraged to give gifts as an expression of how they feel about the people in their lives. While material items represent an exchange of emotions with someone we love, children also learn the value of sharing and giving and receiving by doing kind things for each other, sharing their spirits and souls with each other.

A healthy heart chakra is one that learns an effective balance between giving and receiving. If you were encouraged to share yourself with others, were you also encouraged to receive gifts in gratitude? So often in our culture, we are taught to refuse gifts out of politeness, to deny the offering of a friend to pay for a meal. Giving is deemed virtuous, but taking is deemed greedy. But when denied the opportunity to receive, you may eventually give so much that you are left with nothing in return and then suffer the consequences of scarcity. What are your values of giving and receiving? What do you share with others? When do you allow or disallow others to give to you? What did the adults in your life teach you about giving a receiving when you were in grade school?

Romance

Grade school is the age when puppy love buds into childhood romance. Children start to feel the emotions of connection with others, and the desire to share that love romantically. Did you have a childhood romance? Did you suffer rejection at the hands of grade school crush? Were you the recipient of romantic gestures? Did you welcome those advances, or deny them?

Ecological Element - Air

The element for the heart chakra is AIR, symbolic of space, freedom, expansion, and openness. Breath is life, and air is the vehicle for breath to move through the body and provide life. Air is invisible, and we breathe it everyday, symbolic of all the invisible things we carry with us through our lives: our thoughts, our passions, our feelings, our spirits, and our minds.

Breath

An old folklore that is often studied by scientists and chemistry students is the concept that at any given moment you are breathing the same air as Caesar's dying breath. Caesar's last exhaled breath is one liter of air that consists of approximately 10^{22} molecules which has been mixed up in the earth's atmosphere over two thousand years. Assuming that exhales has been evenly distributed through the world over the two thousand plus years since Caesar died, you can surmise that one of the molecules you just inhaled was exhaled by Caesar during his dying moments. In essence, at any given moment, every breath you take you are inhaling the same molecules that have been exhaled by others. You are constantly sharing air with everyone else who has ever roamed the planet.

Thus, the element of air, through the vehicle of our breath, is symbolic of the basic human connection that we share with every living being on the planet, the experience of life. We are all made of the same stuff, and that stuff needs to the breath of air to survive and live the human experience. Understandably then, air represents our ability to relate to anyone and to be able to feel compassion.

Flight

Whether it be airplanes, helicopters, parasailing, hang-gliding, sky-diving, zip-lining, kite-flying, or hot-air-ballooning, people have developed a multitude of modalities to simulate the concept of flying in the clouds like the birds. To escape from the grip of gravity, weightlessness, if even momentarily, provides a sense of freedom and lightness to the human experience. With freedom comes a release from the sensations of burden and responsibilities that plague most people. Flight of any kind is a way to, at least momentarily, take the weight of the world off your shoulders and feel weightless and carefree.

Emotional Balance - Love & Grief

A healthy and balanced heart chakra manifests in a healthy relationship with love and grief in your life.

The light emotion of the heart chakra is love. It governs all things in our lives that surround the concepts of relationships, connection, compassion, and humanity. A balanced heart chakra supports healthy boundaries in relationship as well as a healthy level of intimacy.

The shadow of the core chakra is grief. Grief is the emotion of loss and emptiness and is often related to sadness, depression, loneliness, abandonment, and rejection. Ironically, it usually manifests in the body as a very dense and heavy sensation.

Characteristics of Imbalance

Excessive Heart Chakra

An excessive heart chakra means too much energy in the heart, too much focus on staying connected and maintaining relationships. This is often a result of fear of loss. Symptoms may include:

neediness
co-dependency
smothering and coddling others in relationship
asthma & other breathing issues
breast cancer
difficulty receiving from others
feelings of rejection
depression
sadness

When women take care of others without taking care of themselves, putting the needs of others far above their own, giving more than they receive, they often end up battling breast cancer. The illness forces them to depend on others and learn how to let other care for them. They are forced to learn how to receive. Thus, breast cancer is a common result of an excessive heart chakra, an imbalance in giving and receiving.

Deficient Heart Chakra

A deficient heart chakra is lacking energy in the areas of love, compassion, relationships, and giving. Symptoms may include:
loneliness
extreme introversion
aloofness
lack of intimacy
heart disease
isolation
difficulty sharing or giving to others
difficulty breathing, particularly exhalations
heart attack

When people put materialism and success ahead of human compassion and end up being cold and harsh in a dog eat dog world, it is as if their hearts shut off and they become unfeeling in the name of success. Physically, this may eventually manifest in heart disease, or even heart attack, the complete shutting off of the heart, an inability to pump love through your system.

Extreme Heart Chakra

An extreme heart chakra means that energy shifts from giving to taking, compassionate to cold, depending upon the situation and circumstance at hand.
neediness coupled with isolation
emotional unavailablity
difficulty maintaining intimate relationships

Heart Chakra Dominance

A dominant heart chakra means that you have particular skill and talent in the areas of love, compassion, relationship, and connection. These individuals have an innate ability to nurture others. Careers that are heart chakra dominant include:

nurses
health-care workers
massage therapists
social workers
therapists

Life Lessons - Relate to Others

Aesop's Fable

The Belly and the Members

One fine day it occurred to the Members of the Body that they were doing all the work and the Belly was having all the food. So they held a meeting, and after a long discussion, decided to strike work till the Belly consented to takes its proper share of the work. So for a day or two, the Hands refused to take the food, the Mouth refused to receive it, and the Teeth had no work to do. But after a day or two the Members began to find that they themselves were not in very active condition: the Hands could hardly move, and the Mouth was all parched and dry, while the Legs were unable to support the rest. So thus they found that even the Belly in its dull quiet way was doing necessary work for the Body, and that all must work together or the Body will go to pieces.

In this story, the Members of the Body decide that they are individual pieces, rather than parts of the whole. When they go on strike, they eventually realize the necessity of valuing each individual's role in the functioning of the whole. In order to function in community, one must recognize the interconnected nature of all things, and value the role that each individual plays to contribute to the whole. Thus, relating to others, as the Belly and its Members needed to do to maintain optimal functioning of the whole, is a necessary skill.

The skill of relating to others is governed by the heart chakra. When your heart chakra is balanced, you are able to appreciate the contributions of other individuals to the higher purpose of the whole. When you can relate to where others are coming from, you can value their contributions and appreciate them for their situations. In the case of the body and its members, if one body part is injured or hurt, more than likely another body part will compensate as necessary to maintain function until the injured or ailing part can return to full capacity. The same happens within community and in relationships. A healthy relationship is not necessarily one that is balanced all the time, but one in which the members compensate for each other as necessary. It's an even give and take. When one person needs, another one gives, knowing that eventually, what goes around comes around. Should you need it, when you cannot give and need to receive, someone will be there to give back to you.

Balancing Practices & Prescriptions

Diet & Nutrition

A **deficient heart chakra** is lacking in compassion and love. When any infant (human or animal) is born, mother's milk is the most nourishing and nurturing substance that the infant can receive. Dairy foods symbolic of compassion and love and provide physical and energetic nourishment to your heart chakra. Yogurt, particularly the greek yogurts, also contain live probiotics that help keep the balance of yeasts and healthy bacterias in your system. Milk is very nurturing and loving, so healthy dairy foods (in moderation of course) can support a deficient heart chakra.

Since an **excessive heart chakra** often manifests smothering and co-dependency, the spacious air of leafy greens support the excessive heart chakra as equally as they do for the deficient heart. Including more kale, arugula, spring greens, endive, broccoli, swiss chard, spinach, and collard greens, can lighten the load of any heavy burdens that result from smothering and co-dependency. Women diagnosed with breast cancer are often instructed from holistic health care professionals to drink "green smoothies" as a means of infusing more leafy greens into their diets to support their physical needs, especially during the treacherous processes of chemotherapy and radiation. Beautifully, these leafy greens provide nourishment both physically and energetically.

The **extreme heart chakra** is really the manifestation of an imbalance of giving and receiving, giving all you have which results in neediness, so then taking all you can get. Such imbalance is usually the result of an inability to energetically process love in your system appropriately. Nothing cures the ailing of the heart better than good old-fashioned home cooking. The best way to balance an extreme heart chakra is to learn how to cook, how to love and appreciate the energetic qualities of food from someone who cooks food with love. Sign up for some cooking classes with someone who cooks with love (a loving family member or friend is best) and take the time to learn how to infuse love into your food as you prepare it. Eliminate take-out and dining out and learn to love yourself by preparing healthy loving nourishing food for yourself.

Body Mechanics - Heart Embrace

When you inhale, air is transported through the tubes of your mouth and nose through smaller bronchial tubes into even smaller tubes inside your lungs. These tubes keep branching smaller and smaller like the branches of a tree until eventually, the air is broken down to its smallest form and can be funneled into your heart and added to the blood. From there, your heart pumps the oxygenated blood through arteries to smaller tubes of blood vessels to even the smallest tubes of the capillaries. Think of this entire system of tubes like a massive plumbing system of your body. In plumbing, the pipes should be both solid and pliable in order to best transport their contents. If the pipes are too flexible, they easily collapse, if they are too rigid, they easily break. At the same time, you don't want blockages to form inside the channels either, yet you want the walls of the channels to be thick enough that the contents don't seep out. You also want the contents that are transported through the tubes to be the right temperature and consistency as well. Too cold could make the contents too dense and move too slowly, whereas too hot could make the contents too thin and move too quickly.

A simple easy way to keep the tubes of your respiratory and circulatory system in optimal shape is to first align your chest and ribs in a way that doesn't impinge on the largest of the tubes, and then to breathe air through those open channels. The deeper you breathe, the more the tubes can open. When the heart and lungs exchange air and blood through the system on the physical level, the heart chakra allows the flow of all things in life to work in a relationship of balancing give and take. The flow of your breath is symbolic to the flow of energy through your system. To manage this give and receive of air and blood through your system is to manage the give and receive of energy through your system.

The heart embrace is an exercise that opens the tubes of your respiratory and cardiovascular systems and push air through.

1. Sit up tall and take a deep breath. Take note of the volume, density, and fullness of your breath.
2. Put your thumbs in your armpits and lift your shoulders up towards your ears. This action pulls your shoulder girdle up off your ribcage.
3. Keeping your elbows out to the side, pull them back towards the wall behind you. This action flattens your shoulder blades across your back.
4. Drop your elbows and shoulders down away from your ears, lightly placing your shoulder girdle back into place, more appropriately aligned on your ribcage.
5. Release your thumbs from your armpits and take another deep breath. Take note of the volume, density, and fullness of your breath.

Chances are, your second breath, after you've aligned your shoulder girdle, is fuller than your first. What you have done is released any tension and pressure from your shoulders off of your ribcage, allowing the ribs to have fuller range of motion to provide the most space for the heart and lungs to do their work.

Anytime you feel like you are not giving or receiving appropriately, you are challenged in relationship, or you feel like you can't get a full inhale or exhale, try doing this simple heart embrace exercise.

Exercise

Cardiovascular exercise such as walking, running, biking, stair-climbing, elliptical machines, and other forms of exercise that elevate the heart rate and increase the breath rate are very supportive of the heart chakra. These exercises exercise the muscles of your heart and lungs to function at their optimal ability.

Breathing Practice - Stop & Breathe

To expand your lung capacity and learn to control your breathing is to gain better awareness of your heart chakra and balance it. Therefore, any breathing practice is healing and helpful for the heart chakra. A good way to implement a regular breathing practice into your life is to apply a "Stop-Breathe" consistency to your life. In other words, anytime you find yourself stopping or waiting, at a stop light, waiting in line, waiting on hold on the phone, waiting for your computer to load, etc., use that time to take a deep full breath. Do not start whatever action is next until the full breath is complete. Every deep breath you take sends messages to your brain to relax, slow down, and calm your system. This will result in a slower heart rate, lowered blood pressure, and a calmer state of being. On an energetic level, deeper breaths expand your lung capacity, and fill up your heart with more compassion and love, making more space in your life for deeper relationships and connections with others.

You can do many little things throughout your day to remind yourself of the connection between breath and life.

- While driving, every time you come to a stop sign or stoplight, take a deep breath.
- Match your breath to your steps while walking.
- Take 5-10 deep breaths whenever washing your hands.

- When you are having difficulty relaxing or sleeping, trying counting your breath, evening your inhales to your exhales, 4-6 counts in and out.
- When you feel anxious, nervous, panicky, angry, frustrated, or fearful, take 3-5 deep breaths with your eyes closed and notice how quickly your mood softens.

Elemental Practices – Air

Air, particularly in the form of wind, is the great reminder of the spaciousness of the universe. To connect with and appreciate the power and capacity of air is to recognize the value of space and openness in your life.

Deep Breathing

The absolute best way to bring spaciousness into your life and world is to bring it into your body through deep breathing. While many programs and trainings offer various techniques for effective breathing, it really isn't that complicated. Breathe. Just Breathe. Breathe big, as often as possible. Anytime you feel constricted, limited, tied, or stuck, deep breaths can open the space for you to see more clearly and have more room.

Birds & Feathers

Birds, especially eagles, are viewed as symbols of freedom for their ability to soar high into the sky. Visiting an aviary, bird watching, or feather collecting are all hobbies that can help you connect with freedom through the symbolic magic of birds and feathers.

Wind

Interacting with wind and air has always been a thrill for humanity. From flying a kite to sky-diving, there are many ways to enjoy the adventures of space and freedom through the wind and the air. Next time you go to an amusement park, try a ride that blows the wind through your hair and take a moment during the ride to consciously appreciate the freedom you feel. Find a child and play with a kite while you consciously contemplate the power of air to create space and freedom. Next time you get on an airplane, close your eyes as you take off and feel the wind lift the plane, and then look out the window as you soar above clouds and contemplate the vastness of the atmosphere. Or, simply lay in the grass and stare up at the sky, the clouds and/or the stars and breathe in the fullness of the universe as you enjoy the space above you.

Mindful Concentration Techniques

The following prescriptions are more spiritually based practices that are balancing and healing for the heart chakra.

- Meditating on the color GREEN

- Offering gratitude to AIR

- Visualizing AIR flowing through your whole body as you breathe

- Breathing practices

Journaling Topics

1. What challenges have you faced in relationship?
2. Do you struggle with loneliness or depression, isolation, or lack of intimacy? Where in your life have you felt rejected, and has that affected your ability to love yourself?
3. What is your relationship with giving and receiving? How do you allow others to give to you? When do you deny yourself of gifts being offered to you?
4. Do you have difficulty feeling compassion for others, empathy? What can you do to put yourself in someone else's shoes as a means of understanding the human experiences they are having and how you can relate?
5. Do you have difficulty with your heart, lungs, breasts, or tightness in your shoulders and upper back? What burdens and responsibilities for others do you carry in your shoulders that are not really your burden to bear?
6. Do you have difficulty letting go because you have experienced great loss in your life in the past? How can you grieve and mourn to get through the loss and move on to new space in your life?
7. What losses have you suffered in your life that you have not completely healed from? What great loves have you had in your life that you are grateful for? Are there any great loves that are also losses that you have completely let go of and moved on from?

CHAPTER 8

The Throat Chakra

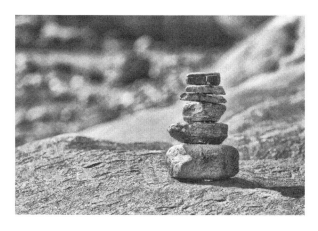

Sanskrit - Vishuddha

Vis = Complete
Suddha = Pure, Absolute

Definition

The vissudha chakra is the center of complete clarity, absolute purity. Vis translates to complete, or spread throughout, and suddha translates to pure, clean, honest, virtuous, clear. Thus, the vissudha chakra is about expression of your being as completely honest, pure, authentic, genuine, clear, and pure.

Governing Realm - Communication

Voice
Language
Music
Communication
Expression
Speaking
Listening

The power of the throat chakra is Communication, governing expression and language, your ability to say what you feel and share what you know. A balanced throat chakra supports effective communication where you are able to say what you mean and others are able to receive your message as it was intended. Furthermore, a balanced throat chakra is able to discern between what is best shared and said and what is best kept silent and secret.

The throat chakra governs our ability to communicate and express ourselves in the world. Just as our throats house vocal chords that vibrate by the pressure of air passing over them, many things outside our bodies function similarly, such as the strings of musical instruments like guitars, pianos, and cellos. Telephone wires, made of mineral, are used to transmit vibrations of sound over large distances. As technology has evolved, so has our ability to share information through computers and the world wide web. Communication is no longer limited to vibrations over wires, but is processed by complex languages inside computer chips and hard drives.

When the throat chakra is balanced, you are able to express your intentions and thoughts clearly without misinterpretation. Issues of ideas being lost in translation or words and language being insufficient to express feelings and emotions are overcome by the energetic vibration emanating from the throat chakra. Artists, writers, speakers, musicians, and entertainers are particularly talented in using the instrument of their throat chakra.

Body Location – Neck & Jaw

The body parts connected to the Throat Chakra are the Neck & Mouth, including your neck, cervical spine, jaw, teeth, tongue, and throat. Your neck provides you with the ability to rotate and twist and turn and look up and look down so that you can have a greater perspective and a wider view of the world. While we want the flexibility, too much flexibility can also be harmful.

Because the cervical spine, the seven vertebrae between the skull and the ribcage, is so flexible, it is easy to cut off the energy flow between your head and the body by misaligning your neck. If you spend a lot of time at a computer screen, sitting at a desk, or even driving in a car, it is likely that you tend to lean your head slightly forward on your neck in order to bring your face closer to the action. Your head is a like a heavy bowling ball. If you balance it evenly atop your spine, there is little effort and muscular energy required to support it. However, if you tend to hold your neck forward, it pulls on your spine, and that weight puts tension on your neck and shoulders and the muscles that support your spine. This is why the muscles around the neck and shoulders often get tight, and why people tend to say that they carry their stress in their neck and shoulders.

Development Stage – Middle School

The throat chakra develops during the middle school years, what is often called the "tween" years. From age ten to thirteen, children are going through puberty, some major changes in their physiology and thus also their energy.

Relationships

Middle School is often the age that children start having puppy love romances. As they go through puberty, the hormones in their systems start to awaken the desire for romance, going beyond the unconditional love of the heart chakra, but more based on mutual interests and intellectual communication as well as physical attraction. Romantic relationships develop and mature based on communication, both verbal and non-verbal, as well as body language and expression. Children at this age, although experiencing the awkwardness of puberty, are much more coordinated with using their bodies and thus much more expressive in their non-verbal communication.

Music

Middle School is often when children are invited to join the school band, orchestra or choir. These classes and school organizations support the function of the throat chakra as they provide a means for children to communicate in ways other than purely verbal expression. At this age, children are starting to develop more individualized musical tastes, and if they choose to play a musical instrument, they can learn to communicate within a group like a band or orchestra.

Sports & Fitness

Middle School is also the age at which sports and other physical activities are encouraged through after school sports and functions. Whether it be dance club or track or football, children are invited to participate in a sport or function that requires physical expression as an individual in part of a team. While children may be on pee wee leagues earlier, it is in middle school when sports really develop a competitive edge to their programming, and students need to find ways to express themselves with their bodies more adeptly

Ecological Element - Mineral

The element for the throat chakra is MINERAL, including stone, metal, and bone. Mineral is the element that most effectively conducts sound. Wires made of mineral are used in telecommunications and computers. Musical instruments often use strings of metal or mineral to produce sound.

Archeology

When archeologists study the ruins of a site, mineral is the element that remains after centuries, thus it is the mineral that they study to determine information about the culture that lived in the region. They can learn a vast amount of information about the culture and people that lived in an area by studying the bones, shards of pottery, and metal tools that remain in the soil. Mineral is the element of information.

When people die, the bones are the one part of the body that doesn't completely decay or get eaten or composted into the soil. The popular forensic science television shows of today illustrate that the study of the mineral of the bones can determine many pieces of information about the life of the person.

Ancestry

While our DNA exists in every cell of the human body, we often refer to our ancestry as living in our blood and bones. Symbolically, as our bones live on long after our death, the bones of the body represent the legacy of our ancestry. In fact, the bones of various holy men are often kept in sacred crypts and considered relics of the church because they hold the DNA code of the saint.

Emotional Balance – Truth & Lies

While many of the morals of Aesop's teach that honesty is always the best policy, lying is common and human. Some psychological studies have shown that people lie an average of three times during the course of a ten minute conversation. We tell lies for many reasons, to impress others, to protect ourselves from possible consequences, to avoid causing pain to someone else, or even to support the potential of a surprise. While some lies are considered "white lies" which are not really harmful, other lies are often considered criminal. Sometimes telling the truth, but failing to share the full story is even considered lying by omission. The balance of the throat chakra comes with the ability to discern when it is appropriate to express, to provide information, and when it is appropriate to repress, to keep information to ourselves.

The light emotion of the throat chakra is expression, the desire to share and give out and to communicate with others.

The shadow of the throat chakra is repression, the desire to keep secret, to hold in, to keep something protected in inside.

A balanced throat chakra is one where you are able to discern when it is best to share, to express, and when it is best to repress, to hold back. We have all met people who tell us too much information, and we have all met people who do not provide enough information. The balanced throat chakra is able to communicate the essential information in the most effective way.

Characteristics of Imbalance

Excessive Throat Chakra

An excessive throat chakra means too much energy in the throat, too much focus on expression and communication. Symptoms may include:

interrupting others
loud-talking
excessive clearing of the throat
over-taking conversations
not allowing others to share or speak
raspy or deep voice
inability or difficulty hearing others

whiplash
laryngitis from over-talking
nodes on the larynx or vocal chords
throat cancer

The person with an excessive throat chakra is rather stereotypical. He enters a room and lets everyone know that he has arrived. His body language takes up more space that his physical stature, and his voices echoes so loudly off the walls that many conversations stop to see who has entered. When involved in conversation with this person, he interrupts, talks for long durations, and brings up a variety of subjects without ever allowing a space for someone else to speak.

Deficient Throat Chakra

A deficient throat chakra is lacking energy in the areas of communication and expression and information Symptoms may include:
> tightness in the jaw or pain from TMJ
> sensitive teeth
> shy or quiet voice
> difficulty speaking up
> high-pitched voice
> shyness
> closed body language or small stature
> sore throats or lumps in the throat

The person with a deficient throat chakra is someone who has a difficult time expressing how they feel. While they may have ideas and awesome creativity, their ability to communicate their ideas to the world is hindered. They have difficulty answering questions and they speak in very short sentences and provide very little information.

Extreme Throat Chakra

An extreme throat chakra means that energy shifts from expressing to repressing, sharing to keeping secrets, loud to quiet, exuberant to shy depending upon the situation and circumstance at hand.

> Over-talkative in familiar settings
> Excessively shy in new surroundings

Throat Chakra Dominance

A dominant throat chakra means that you have particular skill and talent in the areas of communication, expression, and information processing. These individuals have an innate ability to process and communication information. Careers that are throat chakra dominant include:

> public speakers
> motivational speakers
> teachers
> talk therapy practicitioners
> poetry slam artists
> singers
> musicians

Life Lessons – Speak your Truth

Aesop's Fable

The Woodman and His Axe

A woodman lost his axe in the river when it glanced off a tree he was felling. Mercury (the God of Communication) appeared while the man was lamenting his loss. On hearing his tale, Mercury dived into the river, and recovered a golden axe. "That's not mine," said the woodman, so mercury returned it to the river, resurfacing this time with a silver axe. "That's not mine," again said the woodman, and again

Mercury returned it to the river, resurfacing this time with the woodman's own axe. "That's mine," said the grateful woodman. Mercury promptly rewarded the man for his honesty by giving him the golden and the silver axes as well. On hearing the woodman's tale, an envious friend set out to do as the woodman had done, visiting the same spot and deliberately losing his axe in the river. Just as before, Mercury appeared and dived in to recover the lost axe. When Mercury produced a golden axe, the man greedily stretched out for it claiming, "That's mine." Mercury, not pleased with the man's dishonesty, held onto the golden axe and refused to recover the original.

In this story, the woodman speaks his truth to Mercury, and is rewarded for his honesty. Mercury is the Roman God of Communication, the Messenger God, and in this story he rewards he who speaks his honest truth and punishes he who is dishonest. As the Sanskrit name for the throat chakra, *visshuda*, translates to mean "honest purity" this story is an example of how honest purity in the form of communication is a virtue of life. In fact, honesty is such an important policy in life that Aesop wrote many famous fables about speaking truth, the most popular of which is the story of the little boy who cried wolf. The moral of that fable being that those who lie are not believed even when they do speak the truth.

These fables and the concept of honest purity are emphasized in spiritual scriptures of both the Bible and the Yoga Sutras. *Thou shalt not bear false witness* is one of the ten commandments in the Bible, and *satya*, non-lying, is one of the moral restraints (*yamas*) in The Yoga Sutras. Put simply, honesty is always the best policy.

Balancing Practices & Prescriptions

Diet & Nutrition

The **deficient throat chakra** is a quiet throat chakra, one that represses, holds back, and doesn't share. Quite often, those who experience deficient throat chakras are embarrassed or ashamed by the noises that result from eating. To counter this, eat noisy food, and allow yourself to make noises as you eat. Crunchy foods like carrots and celery, chips, and nuts work the muscles of your jaw and tongue and thus work the energetic muscles of the deficient and repressive throat chakra.

In many cultures a good loud belch is considered a compliment to the chef. From a physical perspective, a good belch is a means of letting go of the excess air in the food that your body doesn't need, same goes for flatulence. Many cultures are so ashamed and squelched by farting, mainly because of the sulfuric smells associated with it. However, farting is human and healthy and a necessary physical function of the digestive system. While you may not want to let one rip in an elevator, try eating some broccoli or eggs at home and then as ten year old boys do for fun, celebrate the noises and sounds that emit from your body as a result.

The **excessive throat chakra** is often the result of an over-worked mouth and jaw, so eating foods that require less effort on the part of your teeth is helpful. Try "pre-chewing" your food by cutting it into smaller pieces, or even grinding it up into smoothies or soups. Softer foods that need less mastication and go down quietly can give your teeth and jaw a break and teach you to enjoy the silence. Also, taking more time between your bites and enjoying the silence and stillness that occurs in the moment between the moments can help you learn to hold back and relax.

The **extreme throat chakra** is confused about when to speak up and when to be silent. While many doctors and nutritionists may advocate vitamin and mineral supplements that physically would balance the mineral levels of an extreme throat chakra, an energetic approach would be to eat a wide variety of foods with varying textures and densities to work your teeth and jaws and all different levels. The more different ways you physically learn to work your jaw and tongue and throat, more different ways your throat chakra can adapt to situations in your life.

Body Mechanics – Neck Embrace

There's an old saying that the furthest distance you will ever have to travel is the fifteen inches between your head and your heard. Your neck is the column that connects your head to your body, more specifically, it is the channel between your head and your heart. If thre is a blockage or a kink in this channel (like a kink in your neck) your ability to connect your thoughts to your emotions, your head to your heart, is greatly impacted.

Furthermore, your head is like a large bowling ball of weight that is balanced atop your spine. If your neck is aligned nicely, the weight of this 'bowling ball' balances evenly and almost effortlessly atop your spine. However, if your neck is not in alignment, the weight of your head can pull on your spine, causing neck, shoulder, and upper back tension. The more your neck is out of alignment with your skull, the more weight and pressure you put on the muscles of your shoulders and upper back from the extra pressure of your bowling ball head.

The last of the "embraces" that aligns the chakras in the body is the neck embrace, which is a simple alignment practice that places the bowling ball of your skull neatly into alignment with the column of your neck and spine.

1. Sit up tall, take a deep breath, and say a loud resonant "AHHHHH." Take note of the depth, volume, density, and resonance of the sound and how it feels coming out of your body.

2. Place your index finger on your chin and tuck your chin in ever so slightly, so that your chin is parallel to the floor. In other words, tuck in your chin so that you are not putting your nose where it doesn't belong.

3. Keeping your chin in place, pull the back of you head back, as if you are aligning it along a wall or headrest. Better yet, try this whole exercise while standing up against a wall, or sitting in a high backed chair where your head will hit behind you (ladies, take out your ponytails).

4. Keeping your chin tucked and the back of your head back, lift the crown of your head toward the ceiling. This action will lengthen the space between your earlobes and your shoulder tips.

5. Take a deep breath and say "AHHHH" again. Take note of the depth, volume, density, and resonance of the sound and how it feels coming out of your body.

Chances are, the sound is fuller, louder, longer, deeper, and more vibrant. Anytime you feel like you want to speak more from your center, or you want to share your true feelings, or you just need to connect your head with your heart in more clear communication, try this simple neck alignment exercise.

Exercise

Any exercise that promotes healthy bone density is good for the throat chakra because the bones are the element of mineral. Weight lifting is a great form of exercise to promote the throat chakra because it requires a solid understanding of architecture and alignment, stacking the bones and hugging the muscles into the bones. It also improves bone density and prevents osteoporosis.

Musicians, public speakers, and singers often perform facial exercises in preparation for their performances. Stretching and exercising the muscles around your jaw and mouth can help your throat chakra. Studies have shown that facial expressions are not only a sign of a particular emotion or mood, but they also contribute to that feeling. Furthermore, facial expressions are contagious. For example, if you see someone smiling, you are more likely to respond with a smile than a frown or grimace. Thus, the adage "grin and bear it" has some validity to it because the action of grinning actually puts hormones into your system that will create a sense of happiness, however subtle it may be. So, you might as well "fake it to make it."

Breathing Practice - Bee's & Lion's Breath

Because the throat chakra is directly connected to vibration and sound, adding sound and vibration to your breathing practice can help tune the energies of the throat chakra. To do this, use your thumbs to plug your ears, your middle fingers to lightly close your eyes, your pinky fingers to lightly seal your lips, and gently rest your pointer fingers on your forehead and your ring fingers on your nostrils. Take a deep breath in through your nose, and then exhale through your nose while making a humming sound, like the buzzing of a bee. Throughout the exhalation, feel the vibration echo throughout your skull, perhaps even vibrating your teeth slightly. Take 3-5 breaths like this, and then release your hands from your face and feel the energetic buzz that has resulted.

Another breathing technique that balances communication is called Lion's Breath. The inhaling action treats the excessive throat chakra while the exhaling action treats the deficient throat chakra. Together, the inhale and exhale creates balance. To inhale, squeeze your eyes shut tight and pucker your lips and face, almost like you are sucking on a lemon, and breath in through your nose. To exhale, open your eyes wide while looking up, open your mouth fully and stick out your tongue, exhaling out that back of your throat while vocalizing a loud "HAAA" sound. Do 3-5 rounds of this breath, closing up on the inhale and opening up on the exhale. Then breath 3-5 normal breaths to feel the results.

Elemental Practices – Mineral

Mineral is the densest of all matter, providing the densest capacity to hold information. To connect with mineral is to connect with the deep wisdom and information in your bones.

Hold a Stone

If you are nervous about your need to communicate an important message in a very clear and expressive way, try holding a stone in your hand or wearing a significant stone around your neck to activate the energy of your throat chakra.

Gemology

For centuries, precious gems have been worn as adornment, particularly in the crowns and necklaces of royalty. Each stone has its own qualities and traits that activate different energies, and thus the stones places in jewelry of the monarchs were placed very specifically for the purposes they needed to serve. Nowadays, people study the qualities of various stones and use them for healing purposes, even in the popular practice of hot stone massage. Using crystals or amethysts or other stones for healing is effective not just for the throat charka, but for many energetic ailments.

Chanting or Singing

Using your voice causes vibration through your whole body, and serves to even vibrate your bones from the inside out. Chanting and singing are common practices in many spiritual traditions and religious ceremonies that serve to stir up spiritual energy within your body. Music through singing and chanting often incorporates elements of mineral through musical instruments made of metal (cymbals, bells, stringed instruments, flutes, trumpets, tubas, etc.) that contribute to the vibrations of energy. To sing and to chant is to tune the energy of your body to a different vibration.

Mindful Concentration Techniques

The following prescriptions are more spiritually based practices that are balancing and healing for the throat chakra.

- Meditating on the color BLUE
- Offering gratitude to MINERAL
- Vocal exercises making the sounds of the vowels.
- Chanting and singing practices

Journaling Topics

1. What challenges have you faced in expression and communication?

2. One of the biggest fears people ever face is of public speaking. Do you have difficulty presenting or speaking in front of others or to larger audiences?

3. If you were to pay attention, are your sore throats or times you have lost your voice connected to times in your life when you have had difficulty expressing yourself to others? What areas of your life do you have challenges with speaking your mind?

4. What areas of your life do you find ease in processing information? What areas of your life do you find difficulty in processing information?

5. Do you consider yourself a good listener? Who in your life is a good listener to you? How can you be a better listener, and thus a better communicator in your life?

6. Are the significant relationships in your life challenged by poor communication? What can you do to improve your own communication skills? How can you better express yourself?

7. Do you find yourself interrupting others, or being interrupted by others? Do you find difficulty holding conversations with certain people? How can you improve your end of the conversation?

CHAPTER 9

The Third Eye Chakra

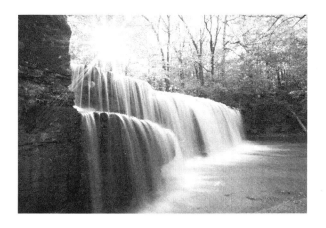

Sanskrit - Ajna

Ajna = Unlimited Power
Ajna = Authority, Command
Ajna = Devoid of Knowledge

Definition

The third eye chakra is the command or authority of the energetic system. Like the brain is the command center of the body, the third eye chakra is the command center of the energetic body. Rather than processing information through analysis, however, the third eye is devoid of analysis, meaning that information is inherently understood, not gained or processed. The third eye functions as intuition.

Governing Realm - Intuition

Wisdom
Knowledge
Insight
Instinct
Intuition
Transformation

The power of the third eye chakra is Intuition, governing wisdom and knowledge, your ability to know and understand your world around you. A balanced third eye chakra supports an ability to take in information from your world and apply it effectively to your own situation.

Intuition is often described as the "still small voice" that whispers the ultimate truth in your inner ear before reason gets involved. If you listen to your intuition, theory is that everything moves smoothly because your first instinct, your intuition, is always right. However, intuition is also rather ungrounded and rarely comes with verifiable proof to support its reasoning. Thus, a balanced third eye chakra is one in which you can trust your instinct, but also effectively apply provable reason and logic to your decisions.

Body Location – Face & Sinus Cavity

The body parts connected to the Third Eye Chakra are those of the face, including the eyes, nose, ears, cheeks, and particularly the forehead. You use your eyes, nose, ears, mouth and skin to bring information into yourself through your five senses: sight, sound, smell, taste, and touch.

While we often refer to the third eye as the space in the center of the forehead that houses the "sixth sense", your intuition. Perhaps a better way to understand it is as the combination of all five senses into one. Physiologically, there is a space in the center of our your skull where the tear ducts of your eyes, the canals of your ears, your nasal passage, and the back of your throat all meet. There are ganglia there for nerve impulses to travel to and from the brain. Thus, when information and stimuli from your eyes, ears, nose, and mouth meet in this place, they combine and send information to the brain to be processed. The first thought, which comes instantly and in a flash that is barely recognizable, is the moment of intuition when these five senses all combine into one. Some indigenous tribes of Africa even encourage their children to try to "smell the sound" or "taste the vision" or "hear the flavor" as a means of teaching them how to develop intuition.

Slight pressure on the forehead touches nerve endings that send messages through to the pineal gland of the brain. This part of your brain, and thus this slight pressure, will tell your parasympathetic nervous system to work, causing your heart rate to slow, your blood pressure to decrease slightly, and your whole body to relax. In relaxation, like in meditation, you can connect deeper inside your mind with yourself, your place of intuition. If you have ever watched a group of children in school taking a test, many of them will hold their non-writing hand on various parts of their forehead, or ever tap their pencils on their heads. This action actually activates the intuitive awareness in the brain and helps better access the information they need to complete the tasks on the test.

Development Stage – High School

The third eye chakra develops in high school, during the teenage years. If you have ever spent any time with teenagers, they are highly instinctual beings, and sometimes act rather arrogantly as "know-it-alls." This is because their third eyes are very active, and they develop into young adults, they are becoming more aware of what works for them and what doesn't.

Ecological Element - Nature

The element for the third eye chakra is NATURE, including plants, animals, and trees. Nature is anything that is alive. Animals are very instinctual and are often able to predict weather patterns and changes in their environment before they appear because they are more in tune with the subtle shifts in the energy, like intuition. Plants and trees don't even have brains to process information, but are constantly cycling energy through themselves and are able to adapt and adjust to circumstances in their environment, especially since they are unable to move from their rooted homes.

Emotional Balance – Reason & Intuition

The human brain is separated into two hemispheres. The right hemisphere governs the creative and intuitive functions while the left hemisphere governs the logical and reasoning functions. Ultimately, we need to balance the creative brain with the logical brain and be able to access either depending upon what we are dealing with in the moment.

The light emotion of the third eye chakra is intuition, as supported by the creative brain, the ability to think outside the box, to use one's imagination, and to be creative.

The shadow of the third eye chakra is logic, the ability to apply reason and analysis to circumstances, to draw upon prior knowledge and apply logic to situations we encounter.

A balanced third eye chakra is one where you are able to be creative and use your imagination but also to be able to ground those lofty ideas in realistic action through logic and reasoning.

Characteristics of Imbalance

Excessive Third Eye Chakra

While exploration of spiritual realms through shamanic journeying, yogic practices, consulting psychics, and so forth have their value, they can result in excessive third eye characteristics. Symptoms may include:

- flightiness
- ditziness
- ungroundedness
- inability to follow logical progression
- dependency on psychics and/or astrologers
- attention deficit
- inability to complete projects
- big visions without follow-through
- impracticality
- headaches or migraines
- excessive day-dreaming

The person with the excessive third eye chakra could be one who is always consulting psychics, angels, or tarot cards to make decisions. Others who are excessive in the third eye chakra are the extremely creative type who is constantly believing that they will become rich or famous from their work without having the ability to properly market or sell their products.

Deficient Third Eye Chakra

A deficient third eye chakra is lacking energy in the areas of creativity and intuition and instinct. Symptoms may include:

inability to visualize
lack of creativity
headaches or migraines

stuck thinking
hyper-analytical
difficulty adapting to change or evolution

The person with a deficient third eye chakra is doesn't have the ability to trust or believe anything that they cannot prove through science and logic. They are often unable to have a vision beyond the practical and logical or to see potential goals or future possibilities.

Extreme Third Eye Chakra

A person with an extreme third eye chakra is one who trusts and believes in creativity and intuition, but is often left disappointed when what they envision doesn't turn out as they hoped, and then they give up on their creativity and depend solely on logic and reason. They are unable to balance the two sides. They are either all logical or all visionary.

Third Eye Chakra Dominance

A dominant third eye chakra means that you have particular skill and talent in the areas of vision, creativity and intuition, and you are able to make your visions into reality, or you have the practical mindset to hire people to do the busywork of making your visions into reality.

Psychics
Healers
Intuitives
Astrologers
Artists
Entrepreneurs
Visionaries
Creators

Life Lessons - Focus Your Vision

Aesop's Fable

The Ant and the Chrysalis

An Ant nimbly running about in the sunshine in search of food came across a Chrysalis that was very near its time of change. The Chrysalis moved its tail, and thus attracted the attention of the Ant, who then saw for the first time that it was alive. "Poor, pitiable animal!" cried the Ant disdainfully. "What a sad fate is yours! While I can run hither and thither, at my pleasure, and, if I wish, ascend the tallest tree, you lie imprisoned here in your shell, with power only to move a joint or two of your scaly tail." The Chrysalis heard all this, but did not try to make any reply. A few days after, when the Ant passed that way again, nothing but the shell remained. Wondering what had become of its contents, he felt himself suddenly shaded and fanned by the gorgeous wings of a beautiful Butterfly. "Behold in me," said the Butterfly, "your much-pitied friend! Boast now of your powers to run and climb as long as you can get me to listen." So saying, the Butterfly rose in the air, and, borne along and aloft on the summer breeze, was soon lost to the sight of the Ant forever.

"Appearances are deceptive."

In this fable, the ant represents the human left-brain as he is only able to apply logic and reason to his experience with the chrysalis, unable to visualize or imagine the potential of it becoming a butterfly. The butterfly represents the human right-brain, the ability and potential of something to transform into something completely different. In reality the metamorphosis of the caterpillar to the chrysalis to the butterfly is a very logical and scientific process. With the power of the vision in the third eye chakra, almost anything is possible, but science a logic must be applicable. If you look at everything in your life at face value and take it exactly as it appears, you could be missing a much larger potential and possibility. Appearances are deceptive.

Balancing Practices & Prescriptions

Diet & Nutrition

The **deficient third eye chakra** is disconnected from nature, living in a concrete jungle, so to speak, and more plugged into a false world than the natural world. This is common in modern culture as we get more and more caught up in eating the quick pre-packaged meals. The further the food is from its natural state, the less energy it provides to the nature of the third eye chakra. Organic and raw food is supportive to the deficient third eye chakra because it brings you back to your more natural instincts. A great prescription for the extremely deficient third eye chakra would be to go back to the old days of living on a farm, growing your own chickens and butchering and processing them yourself. Unfortunately, in modern culture, this is not an easy prescription to fill. However, growing your own food, or participating in a CSA (community supported agriculture) where you know who grows your food and how it is processed is a nice alternative. Sustainable living and eating locally grown foods are very nourishing for the deficient third eye chakra.

The **excessive third eye chakra** is ungrounded, and is almost always coupled with a deficient root chakra, thus the healing foods are the same. Dense proteins like red meat, poultry, whole grains, root vegetables and nuts. People with excessive third eye chakras tend to gravitate towards vegetarianism because the lighter food aids in the exploration of spiritual realms while denser foods of animal proteins keeps one too grounded to go into dreamier places. Vegetarians who experience symptoms of inability to stay grounded could refer to the diet and nutrition prescription for the deficient root chakra for more.

The **extreme third eye chakra** is one that swings from lofty and airy to dense and heavy, which is very similar to the extreme root chakra. It is common for the extreme third eye chakra to want to keep their food separate on the plate, eat all the light food, and then all the dense food, and don't allow the two to mix. The best dietary prescription for the extreme third eye chakra is to mix it up, and in moderation. In preparing meals, make sure you have a balance of light and dense foods and you combine them in your mouth together. Serve yourself foods with everything mixed up on the plate.

Body Mechanics

You have approximately 43 to 52 muscles in your face. Typically, we use our facial muscles to express emotion, but they are also used to block or open our senses to stimuli. For example, you can use several muscles around your eyes to squint or close your eyes to block out things you don't want to see, or you can pucker up your lips and cheeks as an impulse to certain flavors. Learning to relax your facial muscles and still them can help you be more receptive to the information you are bringing into your system through your senses and thus allow them to process through your intuition (in that space where all the senses merge).

As the facial muscles are used to express emotion, think of every facial muscle fiber as a tiny little channel to transmit the energy of emotion. Emotions have an extremely powerful impact on your experience of life because emotion is energy, and energy is contagious. If you walk into a room and you are happy and everyone else is solemn, likely it won't be long and you are feeling solemn as well. Studies have proven that it is easier for people to smile than frown if they are looking at others who are smiling, and vice versa. This contagious energy works internally as well as externally. For example, if you smile, very soon after, you may feel a sensation of smiling through your body, or a pleasant sensation in the body often produces a smile on your face. Furthermore, a smile will send enzymes and hormones through your system that improve immune functioning, fight depression, and regulate moods. Thus the adage, "fake it 'til you make it" applies to faking a smile in life.

Exercise

Laughter yoga is a relatively new phenomenon that is sweeping the globe. Because laughter activates most of the muscles in your face, the exercise of these muscles send neurological messages into your brain that stimulate your third eye chakra and get you more in tune with your intuition. Although it seems more like a fun activity, laughing has many physical benefits and promotes health and wellness on many levels. Studies have shown that just a few minutes of laughter exercise the abdominal muscles as much as a full workout routine. At the same time, laughter causes 'happy hormones' to spread through your system and promote health on many levels. The shaking and vibrations that come with deep belly laughter can strengthen and exercise muscles throughout the body as well as develop core strength. Whether you attend an organized laughter yoga class or just create avenues in your own life to laugh and laugh often, it is great exercise that promotes health and intuitive development.

Breathing Practice - Oceanic Breath

While we often refer to intuition as a "sixth sense" in essence it is actually the merging of all five of your senses. A breathing practice that promotes the merging of the five senses is the *oceanic breath,* which brings a soothing vibration and sound similar to the sound of the ocean to the space inside your skull where all your five senses meet. To do this, first breathe out your mouth with a slight "ha" sound and feel how the back of your throat vibrates slightly. The result is a breath that seems like it would fog up a mirror. Second, apply that same vibrational feeling and sound to your inhalation. The vibrational and vocal inhale will feel and sound almost like a subtle snore. Once you have figured out how to breathe in and out through your mouth with this subtle vibration and vocalization, try it through your nose, keeping the same vibrational feeling at the back of your nose like you had at the back of your throat. The place that vibrates at the back of your nose and throat is your sinus cavity, where your senses of smell and taste and feeling all meet. If you trace your ear canals and your eye ducts into your skull, you'll find that they meet in that same space as well. For example, when you drink carbonated liquid while you are laughing, you can feel it in your ears and your eyes because these ducts and canals all meet in one place. Take 5-10 deep breaths into this space in the center of your skull, and you will feel this vibration pervade through your entire skull, softly and subtlely calming your system just enough that you can hear the still small voice of intuition that comes from inside yourself, where all your senses merge, your sixth sense.. This breathing technique is sometimes called oceanic breath because the sound it creates inside your skull is similar to the sound of an ocean, or the sound you hear when holding a seashell up to your ear.

Elemental Practices - Nature

Spending time in nature has always been a way to find inner peace and connect with spirit. Whether you're taking a hike in the woods, a walk on the beach, canoeing on a peaceful lake, bird watching, fishing, or hunting, being out in the great outdoors is a means to exercise your third eye chakra and remember the essential nature of your being.

Time in Nature

Hiking, backpacking, canoeing, kayaking, stand-up paddleboarding, boating, mountain climbing, bird watching, hunting, fishing, skiing, snowboarding, running, biking...the possibilities for outdoor recreation are limitless, and arguably the source of great pleasure. Many people believe that time out in nature is their most peaceful times in life. Try making an effort, every single day, to get outside and connect with nature. Like Henry David Thoreau wrote in his memoirs from living on Walden Pond, the wonders of the universe are present in the ant hills, the treetops, and the calling of the birds and insects everywhere, you only need to take the time to notice.

Pets & Plants

If you live in the city, or getting out to raw nature is difficult, bringing nature into your home is a great way to exercise your third eye chakra. Pets, particularly dogs and cats are extremely expressive creatures who communicate through non-verbal expression, forcing you to use your senses rather than intellect. Not only are the exceptional companions, they are extremely in tune with your vibrations as a human being and often anticipate your emotional needs and provide for you. However, pets can be high maintenance, thus taking care of plants can be a nice alternative that can connect you with nature. Plants and animals, or even indoor trees can all remind you of the natural state of beings and how to access your own natural state.

Tree-hugging

Next time you go for a walk, try taking a moment to stop and actually hug a tree. We use the phrase in so many figurative ways, but how often do we actually take the time to wrap our arms around one of these great beings? Try it. Put your heart, your chest, your breast and your belly right up to the tree's trunk and see how it feels. Indigenous tribes often look at trees as the wisest of spiritual beings on the planet, so to put your heart right up next to one is a deeply spiritual experience. No wonder hunters enjoy the silence and solitude of sitting in a tree stand regardless of if they get their kill or not.

Mindful Concentration Techniques

The following prescriptions are more spiritually based practices that are balancing and healing for the third eye chakra.

- Meditating on the color INDIGO
- Offering gratitude to NATURE
- Spending time out in nature
- Observing animals
- Tending to gardens or plants

Journaling Topics

1. When have you felt a pang of intuition, you didn't listen and wished you had?

2. How observant are you to your surroundings? Can you remember the smells, tastes, touches, and sounds of certain places and experiences?

3. Do you have difficult with any of your senses? Such as blurry vision, challenged hearing, difficulty smelling or tasting or numbness in your sense of touch? When do these challenges frustrate you the most? What do you do to compensate? Which senses are more adept for you?

4. What is your relationship with nature and animals? Do you have pets? Do you spend much time in nature? When you, how does it make you feel.

5. Do you consider yourself an intuitive person? Can you apply your intuition to real life situations? Are your insights grounded in reality or do you get lost in imagination?

6. How imaginative are you? Can you make your dreams into realities?

them of their values and beliefs and apply those practices to daily life.

Whether you follow a specific religion, prescribe to certain laws of science, and/or find your deepest connections within yourself and spirit through interactions in nature, contemplating the deeper philosophical questions of life is governed by your crown chakra.

Body Location – Brain & Skull

The body part connected to the Crown Chakra is the head, particularly the brain and your nervous system. Think of your crown chakra like the halo upon your head, a disc of energy that hovers just above your skull.

Like the third eye chakra, the crown chakra is connected to the brain. While the right brain is the creative brain, it is also the side of our brain that can think philosophically and spiritually, outside the box of science and logic and proof, which is governed by the left brain. Together, the two hemispheres of the brain create the whole. Thus, the brain itself is symbolic of the concept of the crown chakra, two sides, science and spirit, merged together into one whole. Like heaven and earth united, the physical and spiritual layered on top of each other, the logical and creative merged. As the name of the crown chakra *sahasrara* which means '*together with the whole*' implies, the two hemispheres of the brain symbolize the duality of life as the yin/yang, the two combining to form one whole.

Development Stage – Adulthood

The crown chakra develops in adulthood. For some, who never have the inclination to contemplate deeper questions of life, it never really completely develops, which isn't necessary for a full life. However, it is common for students in college to make the greater connections between disciplines and to think on a more complex level, which exercises the crown chakra and gets one thinking about the meaning of life on a deeper context.

Ecological Element - Spirit

The element of the crown chakra is SPIRIT, as in alcohol. Yes, liquor. We even call liquor spirit. When we drink liquor or wine or beer, it causes an energetic response in the crown chakra that opens up the channels to spirit world a little wider. Nearly every spiritual tradition in the world uses liquor in some form or another, such as the Christians drinking wine in holy communion as the blood of Christ. In many other traditions, it is custom to pour the first sip of liquor on the ground as an offering to ancestors. And finally, when we offer a toast to someone, we are toasting the spirit.

Those who get addicted to alcohol (spirits) are really craving a connection to the spirit world, which is why the twelve step programs all include a strong spirituality element. "If you work it, it works," meaning that the twelve step program is a committed and consistent practice of connecting with spirit instead of reaching towards alcohol or other substances to offer a false sense of spirituality. Next time you take a drink, take a moment to honor the ancestors and spirit. Offer a simple prayer of gratitude for the connection between spirit world and physical world.

Emotional Balance – Spirituality & Science

For some, spirituality and science, like spirituality and religion, are not separate either. The more advanced studies of quantum physics and teachings of famous scientists such as Isaac Newton and Albert Einstein are also deeply spiritual. The two disciplines can be considered to support each other.

The light emotion of the crown chakra is spirituality, as supported by the creative brain and the ability to think about things and concepts that cannot be proven, but to have a faith and belief and understanding of things outside the realm of practicality and logic.

The shadow of the crown chakra is science, the ability to hypothesize and conduct experiments to prove or disprove theories. In short, the shadow side is "what you see is what you get."

A balanced crown chakra is one where you are able to be think outside of that which can be proven, but also to be able to ground those ideas in practical life.

Characteristics of Imbalance

Excessive Crown Chakra

While prayer and spiritual practice is supportive of a fulfilling life, if one relies too much on surrender to God and Spirit and doesn't take practical action, excessive crown chakra symptoms (which are very similar to excessive third eye chakra symptoms) can result:

* flightiness
* ditziness
* ungroundedness
* inability to follow logical progression
* dependency on prayer
* attention deficit
* inability to complete projects
* big visions without follow-through
* impracticality
* headaches or migraines
* excessive day-dreaming

There is a common story told in churches and spiritual centers around the globe. A man in his home was listening to the radio and heard a warning of a flood coming. Instead of heeding the warning to evacuate his home, he got on his knees and prayed to God to save him. As the floodwaters started to rise, a neighbor came over offering to drive him to safety, but the man said, "I have a strong practice in prayer. God will save me." A couple days later, the floodwaters had risen up to the second level of his home and the man was sitting atop his roof when a helicopter and dropped a ladder for him. He refused, stating again that his prayers to God would save him. Eventually, his home was consumed by the floor, and he drowned. At the gates of Heaven he asked God why his prayer wasn't answered and God said, "I sent you a radio announcement, a helpful neighbor, and a helicopter, each of which you refused. So now, I have saved you by inviting you into the kingdom of Heaven." The moral of this story is that God comes in many forms, you must only open your eyes. However, to receive the gifts of God, you must be grounded enough in the practicalities of earth.

Deficient Crown Chakra

A deficient crown chakra is lacking energy in the areas of faith and belief and spirituality. Symptoms may include:
An excessive "see it to believe it" attitude
inability to visualize
lack of creativity
headaches or migraines
stuck thinking
hyper-analytical
difficulty adapting to change or evolution
poor eye-sight

The person with a deficient crown chakra is doesn't have the ability to trust or believe in anything spiritual or non-physical. While they may go to church and have a religious practice, it is purely out of habit and routine and lacks in true faith.

Extreme Crown Chakra

A person with an extreme crown chakra is one who commits to a consistent practice of prayer and or following a religious or spiritual path, but then feels that prayers go unanswered and swing to complete disbelief. Quite often these individuals were raised in a strict religious path that is steeped heavily in tradition but they do not fully understand the faith behind the practices.

Crown Chakra Dominance

A dominant crown chakra means that you have a deep faith in spirituality and a consistent and applicable practice that supports your belief system. When tragedy or trauma happens in life, a person with a dominant crown chakra is able to tap into their spiritual source and find comfort and even explanation for the difficulties in life. They often serve as counselors or spiritual advisors to others during times of crisis.

Ministers
Priests
Spiritual Teachers
Life Coaches
Inspirational Writers
Gurus
Self-Help Authors

Life Lessons – Set Your Intention

The Fable of Three Trees

Once there were three trees on a hill in the woods. They were discussing their hopes nd reams when the first tree sdaid, "Someday I hope to be a treasure chest. I could be filled with gold, silver and precious gems. I could be decorated with intricate carving and everyone would see the beauty."

Then the second tree said, "Someday I will be a mighty ship. I will take kings and queens across the waters and sail to the corners of the world. Everyone will feel safe in me because of the strength of my hull."

Finally the third tree said, "I want to grow to be the tallest and straightest tree in the forest. People will see me on top of the hill and look up to my branches, and think of the heavens and God and how close to them I am reaching. I will be the greatest tree of all time and people will always remember me."

After a few years, a group of woodsmen came up the trees. When one came to the first tree he said, "this looks like a strong tree, I think I shall be able to sell the wood to a carpenter," and he began cutting it down. The tree was happy because he knew that the carpenter would make him into a treasure chest.

At the second tree a woodsman said, "this looks like a strong tree, I should be able to sell it to a shipyard." And the second tree was happy because he knew he was on his way to becoming a mighty ship.

When the woodsmen came upon the third tree, the tree was frightened because he knew that if they cut him down his dreams would not come true.

One of the woodsman said, "I don't need anything special from my tree, so I'll take this one," and he cut it down.

When the first tree arrived at the carpenters, he was made into feed box for animals. He was then placed in a barn and filled with hay. This was not at all what he had prayed for. The second tree arrived at the shipyard and was made into a small fishing boat, and his dreams of being a mighty ship and carrying kinds and queens had come to an end. The third tree was cut into large pieces and left alone in the dark.

The years went by and the trees forgot about their dreams. Then one day, a man and woman came to the barn. She gave birth and they placed the baby in the hay in the feed box that was made from the first tree. The man wished he could have made a crip for the baby, but this manger would have to do. The tree could feel the importance of this event and knew that it had held the greatest treasure of all time.

Years later, a group of men got into the fishing boat made from the second tree. One of them was tired and went to sleep. While they were out on the water, a great storm arose and the tree didn't think it was strong enough to keep the men safe. The men woke the sleeping man, and he stood and said "peace," and the storm stopped. At this time, the tree knew it had carried the King of Kings.

Finally someone came and got the third tree. It was carried throughout the streets as the people mocked the man carrying it. When they came to a stop, the man was nailed to the tree and raised in the air to die at the top of a hill. When Sunday came, the tree realied it was strong enough to stand at the top of the hill and be as close to God as possible because Jesus had been crucified on it.

Each of the trees got just what they wanted, just not in the way they had imagined. Prayers are always answered.

151

This fable, in reference to Christian spirituality and the stories of Jesus teaches that intentional prayers are always answered, but not necessarily in the manner in which you expect. While the trees set their intentions, they were forced to let go of the exact ways in which those intentions were made into reality. When they surrendered to their fate, their true destiny, based on their prayers, was revealed to them. In truth, what came of their prayers was even greater than they ever could have imagined for themselves.

A balanced crown chakra allows you to set your intention, say your prayer, and then let go of the outcome so that Spirit can make your intention into a reality even greater than you an imagine yourself.

Balancing Practices & Prescriptions

Diet & Nutrition

The **deficient crown chakra** is the result of a lack of connection with spirituality. The dietary prescription for this condition is to drink spirits, alcohol IN MODERATION. The key, however, is not just to drink more alcoholic beverages, but rather to do so in conjunction with a spiritual practice. Almost every religious tradition uses wine in one form or another as a means to connect with Spirit, such as red wine used in communion as a means of drinking the blood of Christ. When alcohol is used to toast and honor and individual and offered as a prayer of that person's humility and sacredness with the divine, it is an infusion of energy to the deficient crown.

Another dietary prescription for the deficient crown is simply to eat less. Too much food results in a density that prohibits exploration of spiritual realms and inhibits connection with Spirit. A diet heavy in red meat and dense foods like root vegetables and heavy grains will weigh you down to worldly and material matters rather than spiritual endeavors. Fasting, is a common practice in religious and spiritual traditions because it promotes spirituality and connection to the divine.

The **excessive crown chakra** is one that lacks grounding, and often manifests in a lack of appetite or forgetting to eat, or when you do eat, it is light foods without much substance. Someone whose head is always in the clouds with an excessive crown chakra needs grounding and bringing back to earth. In addition to just eating more and more often, a diet rich in root vegetables and even some red meat is very grounding.

A common manifestation of an **extreme crown chakra** is heavy eating coupled with excess use of mind-altering substances, such as getting high on marijuana and then getting the munchies. In general, modern culture lives in a constant state of deficient crown chakra, focusing on materialism rather than spiritualism, and the result is a craving of spirituality through inappropriate means like addiction to "spirits" (alcohol and other mind-altering substances). Then too much of those "spirits" results in the body's need to be grounded which expresses itself in the form of hunger. It becomes an insatiable cycle. The treatment, mindful eating, for this is very simple, yet challenging to fulfill because it requires discipline and consistency. Try applying spirituality to your daily life, such as daily morning prayer with your coffee, offering gratitude over your meals, and eating your food as if it is nourishing your spirit and your soul on the same level as it is nourishing your body. Treat your body as the temple that it is and treat your food as the golden relics that you put into that temple.

Body Mechanics

The muscles of your head and skull, unlike those of your face, are not easily moved without external manipulation. However, like the rest of your body, to align your muscles around the energy of the chakras helps exercise the chakras. One great way to exercise the muscles of your head and skull is through cranial sacral therapy. The slight and subtle adjustments of the tissues encasing your skull can have a dramatic effect on the pressure around your brain, thus providing more space and better functioning of your brain. This is probably why a good head massage by your stylist when you get a haircut always feels so good as well. Ironically, we gravitate towards providing ourselves what we need. When people get headaches, they often rub their heads to relieve the pressure. It truly helps. A consistent and daily practice of massaging your skull, manipulating the tissues encasing your skull can help stimulate and exercise and relieve pressure from your crown chakra.

Exercise

In modern culture, people often get too caught up in logic and reason, analysis and process. When this happens, headaches, control issues, and even migraines may result. "Stinking thinking" can quickly devolve into anxiety, panic attacks, depression, fear, rage, or any number of other negative emotions. When you turn yourself upside-down, your head becomes like a salt shaker and drains all those nit-picky thoughts to the ground through the force of gravity. Furthermore, thinking too much is rather difficult when fresh blood and oxygen is flooding your brain from your heart. As an added bonus, when you turn yourself upside-down, it is like turning your world upside-down and you can see things from a whole different perspective, one that uses your creative brain as much as your logical brain.

As we spend most of our day upright, and most of our sleeping time prone, our bodies are not used to going upside-down. For many, there is a huge fear factor involved with turning the body upside-down, particularly because it means taking your feet (your root support) off the ground. However, doing so is highly beneficial to honoring, recognizing and sustaining the cyclical nature of all things. The adage "as above, so below" is injected into the body through the practice of inversions, and thus teaches you to fully engage in the value of Heaven on Earth. Anything that brings your head below your heart will facilitate the physical action of an inversion.

Many religious traditions apply specific bodily movements during prayer as a means of moving energy through the body to connect with Spirit. Protestants kneel, Catholics take the sign of the cross, and Muslims bow on a prayer rug. One way to take your practice of surrendering to Spirit into your life is to offer a specific prayer before, during, and after your physical exercise. You may link specific intentions to each movement, or you may send your prayers and thoughts through your body as you move with intention.

Breathing Practice - Balancing Breath

As your crown chakra is directly connected to your brain, balancing the two hemispheres of your brain to work together will aid in balancing the energy of the crown chakra. Balancing breath through your nostrils can facilitate this process.

When you breathe through your nose, nerves in your nostrils send messages to your brain. Air flow through the right nostril sends messages to the left brain, which is more directly connected with logic and reason. Air flow through the left nostril sends messages to the right brain, which is more directly connected with creativity and imagination. In your natural automatic breathing pattern, one nostril will dominate your breath for about ninety minutes and then the dominance will switch to the other nostril. To find out which nostril is dominant at any give moment, simple hold each nostril closed for a full breath to determine which one is easier to breathe through.

To balance your breath, relax and breathe out completely. Then imagine breathing in through your right nostril, and then out through your left nostril, and then in through your left nostril, and out through your right nostril. Continue for several cycles of breath. On your last round of breath, breathe through both nostrils.

Elemental Practices - Spirit

The best way to connect with and find "just right" in your crown chakra is to develop a consistent and daily spiritual practice. If you prescribe to a particular religion, that may mean finding ways to infuse the rituals of your religion into your daily life. The list below offers other ways to infuse spirituality into your daily life.

Daily Prayer or Devotions

While many people make a practice of prayer when they go to church on a weekly basis, or when they encounter challenge or trauma or tragedy, a consistent and daily practice of prayer and devotion without any specific purpose or need will help bring the crown chakra and your connection to Spirit more in line. Think of prayer as a way to maintain a healthy relationship with Spirit by conversation. You may choose to commit to a practice like those offered from many of using a rosary or mala beads as a means of offering devotions through consistent ritual prayers. Or, you may choose to simply sit down once or twice a day and simply speak from your heart to Spirit, in both requests and gratitude.

Meditation & Contemplation

While prayer is talking to Spirit, meditation is often considered listening to Spirit. While many people consider meditation as a practice in turning off your brain, I prefer to think of meditation as a practice in tuning into the deeper wisdoms that exist inside your thoughts. Taking time each day to simply sit and stare off into space and day-dream is an excellent practice because eventually you learn to pay attention to those thought and often find amazing insights and epiphany moments come out of those moments.

Journaling

One excellent way to converse with the Spirit within yourself is to develop a consistent journaling practice. To sit down and write out your thoughts, about your day, and process your emotions is an excellent way to have a conversation with the deepest parts of yourself. If you commit to writing for a certain amount of time or number of pages everyday, you may find that at a certain point each day as you write, the words start to give you insights to your life and guidance as if you are talking directly to Spirit.

Ancestor Shrine

One excellent way to connect with Spirit is to connect with our ancestors who have left their bodies and joined the spiritual realm. We often think of our ancestors as angels on our shoulders, there to guide us and support us in our journey through life. Having developed and fulfilled a personal relationship with our ancestors when they were alive helps us to relate to them as agents of the Spirit world. If your ancestors were difficult people for you to live with in life, you can think of them in Spirit world as "getting it" now, and thus they have a vested interest in "fixing" what they messed up in life, but they can only do that in partnership with those of us left on earth. Our ancestors in Spirit world cannot work as our agents and angels without our invitation, so prayer and conversation with them is vital. When someone close to us dies, particularly if that death is sudden and tragic, we often create shrines for them composed of photographs, flowers, candles, notes, and other gifts. Their graves become another form of a shrine. A shrine serves as a means to open a sort of spiritual portal through which we can communicate with our ancestors. Why not create a permanent shrine for your ancestors? Replenish it with fresh flowers and gifts on a regular basis. You could even visit this shrine everyday a part of your daily routine. Drink your morning coffee or evening after dinner glass of wine with your ancestors and talk with them as if they are sitting in the room with you. Tell them what you need their support for. Thank them for how they helped you through some challenges. Light a candle each time you visit them. Bring them into your life in a new role now that they are no longer here in the physical.

Mindful Concentration Techniques

The following prescriptions are more spiritually based practices that are balancing and healing for the crown chakra.

* Meditating on the color VIOLET or WHITE

* Keeping a gratitude journal

* Meditation

* Mantra Practice

* Daily Prayer & Devotions

Journaling Topics

1. What were, if any, the spiritual and/or religious practices and traditions followed and offered by your family when you were growing up? How have you continued with those in your life? Which of those practices reside with you?
2. Do you believe in God or Spirit? If yes, where and when do you feel most connected to and supported by this Higher Power?
3. Describe one of those times in your life when you realized or

experienced the ultimate vastness and complete beauty of the universe and the world?

4. When and where do you feel most at peace in your life?

5. What is your relationship with your ancestors? Do you talk with them? How have you or can you facilitate and active partnership with them in your life?

CHAPTER 11

Conclusion

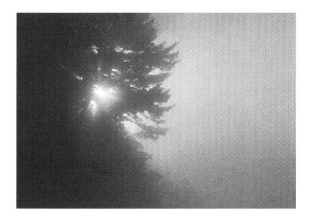

Goldilocks meets Snow-White

"The Story of the Three Bears," which was originally published in 1837 by Robert Southey in a collection of essays and stories called *The Doctor,* bears many similarities to the story "Snow White" published in *Children's and Household Tales* by the Brother's Grimm in 1812. While Goldilocks wanders through the woods to a cottage inhabited by three bears, Snow White wanders through the woods to a cottage inhabited by seven dwarves. Goldilocks tastes porridge, sits in chairs, and sleeps in beds while

Snow White eats bread, drinks wine, and sleeps in beds as well. With this in mind, let's continue our story from Chapter One.

Snow-White

Across the woods in a little cottage similar to that of the three bears, seven dwarves returned home from their work in the mountains to a find a young girl about the same age as Goldilocks asleep in one of their beds. She had hair as black as ebony, cheeks as red as blood, and skin as white as snow. Having seen that she had nibbled from each of their seven loaves of bread, and drunk of each of their seven cups of wine, and tumbled in each of their seven beds, they recognized that this child must have come from a rather distraught situation, so they took care not to wake her.

When Snow-White awoke the next morning, she shared with them her story of being banished by her step-mother, the queen, who was jealous of the young girl's beauty. And so, Snow White stayed with the dwarves, tending house for them as they worked each day in the mountains. They warned her not to let anyone into their cottage while they were away, for fear the queen might find her.

Snow White learned many things from the dwarves over the years, and grew into a beautiful young woman who far-surpassed her evil step-mother queen in beauty and brains. Although the queen did find Snow White and attempted three times to bring young Snow White to her demise, each time, Snow White was able to narrowly escape the hands of death until eventually a prince rescued her from slumber induced by a poisoned apple and brought her back to the kingdom to become his bride. The evil queen recognized her step-daughter and became ill from her envy and died.

While living with the dwarves, Snow White was provided a healthy and stable home. Thus, when the time came for her to be challenged by the outside forces of her step-mother's attempt to kill her, she was able to compensate and eventually find stability again and flourish.

The beauty of this story is that the seven dwarves loved and respected Snow-White for her virtues and gifts instead of looking at them with envy or jealousy or other negative emotions. They allowed her to shine from her inner truth and share with them her strengths. If we look at the Disney version of this fairy tale, each dwarf is named for his personality and characteristics: Sleepy, Happy, Sneezy, Doc, Grumpy, Dopey, and Bashful. Each one is honored and valued for his individual characteristics and their contributions to the community as a whole. Like the seven chakras, each of the dwarves serves his role, contributes to the whole, and respects each other for his identity.

The Power of Seven

That Snow White lived with seven dwarves is symbolic of the seven major energy centers (chakras) of the energetic anatomy system. Because energy is contagious, when Snow-White ate of the seven loaves, drank of the seven goblets and tried each of the seven beds, she was infused with the spiritual healing medicine of the seven loving dwarves.

True balance of the chakras is like functioning in balance within a community. Everyone needs to fulfill their own individual role, and sometimes those roles are called into action more than other times, and sometimes those roles are called to rest more than other times. None of the dwarves are considered *negative*, but rather, each of them holds their own purpose. For example, sometimes sneezes and grumpiness are called for in the moment, while other times happiness and smarts are necessary.

Be Yourself

That Snow White lived with seven dwarves is symbolic of the seven major energy centers (chakras) of the energetic anatomy system. Because energy is contagious, when Snow-White ate of the seven loaves, drank of the seven goblets and tried each of the seven beds, she was infused with the spiritual healing medicine of the seven loving dwarves which helped her to be her most radiant true self.

True balance of the chakras is like functioning in balance within a community. Everyone needs to fulfill their own individual role, and sometimes those roles are called into action more than other times, and sometimes those roles are called to rest more than other times. None of the dwarves are considered *negative*, but rather, each of them holds their own purpose. For example, sometimes sneezes and grumpiness are called for in the moment, while other times happiness and smarts are necessary. Each dwarf was valued for who he was.

Ralph Waldo Emerson once said, "to be yourself in a world that is constantly trying to make you something else is the greatest accomplishment." As the dwarves valued each other for their individuality, you can value yourself for your own individuality by following the prescriptions and guidelines in this book to find "just right" for yourself and be yourself in whatever challenging situations your encounter.

ALSO BY TERI LEIGH

Yoga Roots: An Interactive Guide to the Chakras

Published: August 8, 2012
Print Length: 107 Pages
Size: 327 MB
Type: Interactive Multi-Touch eBook
Available on Mac and iPad through the iTunes store.
$14.99

Through multi-touch interactive images, short videos, audio guided meditations, and artistic nature photography you will learn how to use simple techniques to bring balance into your life anytime and almost anywhere. The practices in this book are based on the practices of yoga, but need not be applied only to yoga.

Yoga Roots: An Elemental Guide to the Chakras

Published: August 27, 2012
Print Length: 84 Pages
Size: 12.9 MB
Type: eBook
Available as PDF download at www.terileigh.com
$6.99

Explore your chakras as they connect and relate to your physical experience. You will learn how to use simple techniques to bring balance into your life anytime and almost anywhere. The practices in this book are based on the practices of yoga, but need not be applied only to yoga. This book is a PDF version of Yoga Roots: An Interactive Guide to the Chakras. It includes all the content from the interactive guide to EXCEPT the multi-touch images, and audio/video elements.

Yoga with TeriLeigh iTunes Podcast

Published: March 2008 - Present
Size: varies
Type: podcast
Available as subscription or download for iTunes podcasts
OR to play directly from www.terileigh.com/podcasts/index
FREE

This yoga practice is for students with a basic understanding of yoga alignment and vinyasa flow. Challenging and spiritual Vinyasa Yoga classes fosters a deeper connection between your physical experience of life and your spiritual awareness. TeriLeigh trained with Baron Baptiste, Sean Corne, Rod Stryker, and more.

Prana Pages Blog

Published: June 2008 - Present
Size: varies
Type: blog
Authors: Teri Leigh & Sandy Krzyzanowski
New posts weekly at www.terileigh.com/blog
FREE

ABOUT THE AUTHOR

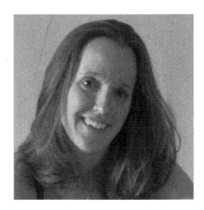

TeriLeigh holds Bachelor's Degrees in Creative Writing and Literary Studies and a Master's Degree in Teaching from Beloit College. With emphasis on clear communication, best practices in education, practical skills application, and effective learning strategies, TeriLeigh has been teaching, speaking, and presenting since 1991. She has experience in teaching the following subjects to a wide variety of audiences: English, communication, public speaking, self-awareness, mindfulness, body mechanics, yoga, yoga instruction, symbolism, and shamanism.